Root Canal Cover-up Exposed! Many Illnesses Result

Dentist to the Stars Discovers Hidden Truth... Tells What to Do

George E. Meinig, D.D.S., F.A.C.D.

Forewards by:
Jeffrey Bland, Ph.D.
Jerome Mittelman, D.D.S., F.A.P.M.

Introduction by:
Edwin C. Van Valey, D.D.S., F.A.C.D., F.I.C.D.
(Past President, American Association of Endodontists

Commentary by:
Lendon H. Smith

Bion Publishing
Ojai, California

Published by Bion Publishing
First Printing 1993

Library of Congress Catalog Card Number 93-72133

Meinig, George E.
Root Canal Cover-up Exposed!
Many Illnesses Result.
Dentist to the Stars Discovers Hidden Truth...Tells What to Do.

Bibliography: P.
Includes index.
1. Publishers and publishing — Handbooks, manuals, etc.

ISBN 0-945196-14-8

Important Notice
Warning and Disclaimer

Although the author and publisher have exhaustively researched all sources to ensure the accuracy and completeness of the information contained in this book, we assume no responsibility for errors, inaccuracies, omissions, or any inconsistencies herein. Any slights of people or organizations are unintentional.

This book is primarily a report about the reams of scientific data published and subsequently buried years ago regarding the exhaustive 25 year root canal research program conducted by Weston A. Price, D.D.S., F.A.C.D. and a group of scientists working under the auspices of the American Dental Association's "Research Institute." The purpose of the book is to alert readers to the possible ill health side effects that were discovered to result from infected teeth, tonsils, and other oral tissues.

Readers of the information and material contained in this book should keep in mind that the various degenerative diseases that were found to take place during these studies also commonly arise from infections, other than those from teeth, and are also commonly due to nutritional deficiencies and/or excesses and to the wide range of biochemical individuality that exists.

Neither the author or the publisher can assume any dental, medical, or legal responsibility in having the contents of this book considered as a prescription for any particular individual or as a direct source of individual dental and/or medical advice.

Action on any question related to medical treatment should be deferred to a physician, as examination and assessment of all of a patient's medical conditions must be taken into consideration in the development of an appropriate diagnosis and treatment plan.

Printed in the United States of America

J.W. Bender, N.D. B.Sc.
22 McDOUGALL RD.
WATERLOO, ONT., N2L 2W5
(519) 885-3720

Root Canal Cover-up Exposed!
Many Illnesses Result

DEDICATION

To my dear wife Eleanor and our family, each of whom has so deeply enriched my life.

To Dr. Weston Price for his unusual abilities and truth seeking dedication to improve the practice of dentistry and the lives of people everywhere.

Happy is he who has to know the reason for things.

– Virgil

ABOUT THE AUTHOR

George E. Meinig, D.D.S., F.A.C.D.

Early in his practice, at a time when few dentists treated root canal infections and only a handful of dental schools gave instructions about the subject, Dr. Meinig practiced root canal therapy and taught the subject at dental association sessions around the middle west.

These professional activities led to his being one of the founding members that started the American Association of Endodontists (root canal therapists).

After World War II service in the air corps, because of this background in root canal therapy and his holistic and nutritional approach to practice, Dr. Meinig was selected to manage the Twentieth Century Fox Studio dental office.

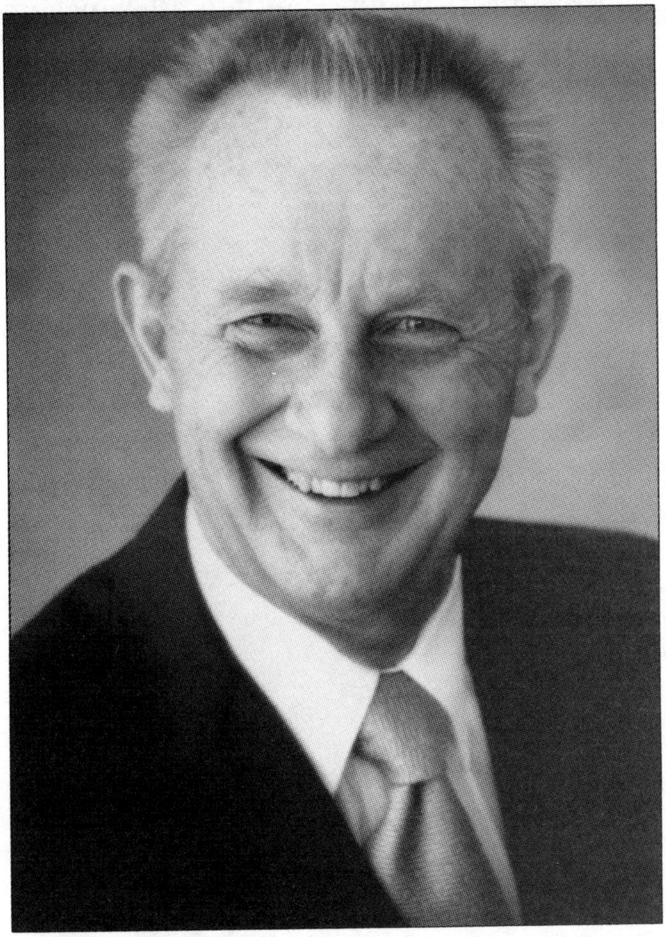

Dr. Geroge E. Meinig

His participation as a member of his dental society's speaker's bureau was a forerunner of lectures he made in many parts of the United States and in four foreign countries.

As a columnist for 17 years, Dr. Meinig's *Nutritionally Speaking* articles appeared weekly in the Ojai Valley News and his book *"NEW"trition — How to Achieve Optimum Health* grew out of that endeavor.

Learning of the meticulous 25 year root canal research of Dr. Weston Price and the serious side effects that can result, Dr. Meinig in consideration of his own opportune, well suited background, found he was anxious about the need for this information to be made public. The thought of the millions of chronic disease sufferers that could be helped was a powerful motivating force.

Along the way, Dr. Meinig has received many recognition citations and awards both nationally and internationally. They include Who's Who in

California, Fellowships in the American College of Dentists, the International College of Applied Nutrition, and the Price Pottenger Nutrition Foundation. From Mexico, he received Certificado de Asistencia and a similar citation from the Federation Dentaire International, Cologne, Germany.

Now retired from his active practice in Ojai, California, Dr. Meinig plans to carry this message about serious side effects of root canal therapy by radio and television appearances, articles in magazines and the press, and with lectures. Through these activities he hopes to stimulate contributions for research about how to sterilize and kill these virulent germs that become locked in the tubules of the tooth's dentin.

Providing of funds that will allow people to save their teeth for a lifetime is a mission of the greatest importance. With all the money that is donated for causes of much less distinction, Dr. Meinig feels their are numbers of individuals out there that will sense what a great opportunity this is for service to mankind.

Table of Contents

FOREWARD

I want to thank you so much for sending on a galley proof copy of your book, Root Canal Cover-up Exposed! Many Disorders Involved. I think this is a most exciting review of the many years of contribution and work you have provided and a nice account of the Dr. Weston Price work from a new, refreshing perspective. I believe as you do that Dr. Weston Price's work has not received the attention and acknowledgement that it deserves. You have put it into a modern context in your book in a "how to" way that can be very helpful in a person making the connection between nutrition, oral health and systemic health.

Please let me know what we can do to help support your efforts to get this message out through your exciting book. My great admiration goes out to you in being honored at the American Association of Endodontists 50th Annual Meeting. That is quite an achievement, to say the least.

Jeffrey S. Bland, Ph.D.
Chief Executive Officer
Healthcomm. Inc.

FOREWARD

Can root canal therapy endanger your health?

Dr. George Meinig writes about research covering thousands of experiments indicating that having root canal therapy could weaken your immune system and lead to serious illness.

Should you have root canal therapy done in your mouth?

Most dentists rely on information they get from the A.D.A. But what if the A.D.A. acts like a trade guild whose main interest is in its members, not you? What if they have been suppressing vital information? What if the information they put out is one-sided?

It seems to us that their actions regarding the controversy over mercury in fillings is a strong indication of this possibility.

Dr. George Meinig has studied the work of Dr. Weston Price, a meticulous researcher. Dr. Price's work shows how germs become trapped in teeth. While dentists fill the root canal, there are still over three miles of inaccessible, untreated tubules from which these germs can pour toxins into your body. These poisons can affect your heart, kidneys, lungs, eyes, stomach, brain, and countless other body tissues. At times, the germs themselves escape into the bloodstream and are carried throughout the body.

Dr. Meinig writes of Dr. Price's twenty-five years of painstaking research, much of it under the auspices of the American Dental Association's Research Institute. He found the results of Dr. Price's research were buried over 70 years ago by non-believers.

We feel that the dental and medical professions will bury the information with demands for further research. Such investigations are necessary, but people should know about Dr. Price's work so that they can decide on their own what is best for them, to make intelligent choices.

By making people aware of the cover-up, Dr. Meinig's exhaustive review of Dr. Price's research will undoubtedly force dentists and physicians to do some "rethinking."

Beyond this, Dr. Meinig describes Dr. Price's research on gum disease and tooth decay in practical terms. This is valuable information. If we don't want to have the dangerous, toxic effects of root canal therapy in our bodies, we can prevent their very need. And here again, Dr. Price helps us make the right choices. We've always said, "If we're not preventing disease, we are preventing health." Dr. Price's work proves it.

Jerome S. Mittelman, D.D.S., F.A.P.M.
Past President International Academy of Nutrition & Preventive Medicine

PREFACE

The public, the dental profession and particularly my fellow members of the American Association of Endodontists (AAE) (root canal therapists) are going to be extremely shocked at my publication of this book and its information about the many side effect disorders that can occur from root canal therapy.

So will the many motion picture greats and other studio personnel I was privileged to serve during my management of the Twentieth Century Fox Studio Dental office. Dr. E. Ray Bronson, who headed the dental office at MGM for many years was asked to establish a similar one in Shirley Temple's former bungalow on the Twentiteth Century Fox lot. Dr. Bronson asked me to handle the day to day practice because of my extensive background in dental procedures, root canal therapy and periodontal gum disease and my interest in nutrition and its prevention attributes. As you can imagine, my associations and experiences at Twentieth Century Fox proved most exciting and valuable. I trust the the information that follows will prove of particular interest and help to the movie industry.

It will, however, be especially difficult for dentists who do root canal therapy and particularly the members of the Endodontic Association to understand my authorship of this data as during their 5-day 50th year annual birthday celebration session in May of 1993, they made a special point of conferring honorary recognition upon me, my brother Dr. Douglas Meinig, a classmate Dr. Henry Kahn and Dr. Saul Levy. We are the last four surviving members of the original 19 founder members that started the root canal organization during a dinner meeting in Dining Room 4 at the Palmer House in Chicago on February 25, 1943.

The public and the dental profession itself for the most part is unaware of the turmoil and difficulties that attended the early years of this organization's existence. During that time there was wholesale extraction of people's teeth and few dental schools taught endodontic (root canal) therapy. In teaching practicing dentists how to save infected teeth we found it difficult to get their attention until we asked, "How could they as dentists ever learn how to save teeth by taking them out?"

That we succeeded in teaching people the value of saving their teeth is no longer a question. The AAE now has almost 4000 members and last year the life of over 24 million teeth was extended by way of root canal therapy.

From the information that follows what is going to blow the minds of dentists and physicians will be learning we have not conquered the problems of focal infection — that infection can be hidden in what are known as the dentin tubules of teeth and also in tonsils. This book in exposing the cover-up facts will point out how bacteria trapped in dentin tubules can escape and be transported to another organ, gland or body tissue where they start a whole new infection.

The dental profession has been very successful in sterilizing root canals and in achieving the healing of large areas of lost infected jaw bone present around teeth. Inasmuch as a large proportion of these teeth remain serviceable for many years it will be exceedingly difficult for dentists to believe such teeth could still be harboring infection.

It is hoped Dr. Stuart Fountain, AAE President and our professional colleagues will not pass hasty judgement or condemnation on my publication of this book. Dr. Fountain's stressing of the importance of the organization's early history and what has been done to save people's teeth was the highlight of that five day 50th anniversary celebration. Not only that but, he introduced each of we founders that were present and all the past presidents and had us sit on the stage while he explained the difficulties of the early years of the Endodontic Association and all it has since accomplished. When Dr. Fountain then asked the 1100 members and their families to rise and applaud all those on the stage for their past efforts, there was hardly a dry eye to be seen.

You will learn the information in this book is not something I have dreamed up but is a review of the most remarkable and momentous 25 year research program conducted about root canal therapy. Not only was the scope of the studies overwhelmingly thorough, but you will learn that it was carried out under the auspices of the American Dental Association's "Research Institute" by dentistry's renowned dental research specialist, Weston A. Price, D.D.S., F.A.C.D.

You will also discover that those 25 years of research were documented by Dr. Price in two volumes totaling 1174 pages and additionally in twenty-five of his 220 scientific articles. Incidentally, this work is available at the American Dental Association library.

It is important at this point for you to know Dr. Price was not alone in carrying out research about the detrimental effects of focal infection but was supported by quite a number of America's outstanding physicians. Just a few of these greats were Charles Mayo, Milton Rosenau, Frank Billings, Ludwig Hektoen, Thomas Forsyth, and Truman Brophy. The contributions of these men and others will be covered in the pages that follow.

You will also learn just how abominable it has been that the solid research of these men was forced underground some 70 years ago by the autocratic opposition of those that did not believe in the focal infection theory.

In the coming pages you will b introduced to the numerous experiments of Dr. Price that disclosed the appalling nature and ability of oral bacteria to make drastic changes in their form and in their activities and just how they become trapped in the dentin tubules of teeth and in the tissues of the tonsils. The shocking surprise turns out to be the way these otherwise friendly oral bacteria mutate and metastasize like the viruses of cancer and therein infect hearts, kidneys, eyes, stomachs, pregnant women and countless other body tissues.

None of you will be any more startled about this information than was I when, a little over a year ago I pursued each and every one of those 1174 pages of Dr. Price's two volume research report. Gradually you will become aware of how our extensive current catastrophic and costly degenerative disease problem significant in this country, to a significant is extent, related to germs that become trapped in dentin tubules of teeth.

There will be a discussion of why this does not mean the end of endodontics and why antibiotics cannot hope to be the answer to the dilemma.

Revealed will be why hearts are the most frequent focal infection attacked organ and how almost all the organs and glands of the body can become involved.

There will be some case histories reviewed and they are accompanied by some 75 photographs. Dr. Price's photographs and x-ray pictures were remarkably good for that period of time but some from other sources are not of comparable quality. Then too, because it was necessary to copy those shown from his two books, in a few instances they are not as clear as we would have liked. I ask your indulgence as I felt your being able to see the magnitude of what is involved made it worthwhile to present all of these pictures.

Although most of the credits for this research are directed toward Dr. Price, it should be recognized that his great, professional team of representatives at the Research Institute do share in all the accomplishments that were disclosed.

Finally, though I expect dentists and other health professionals will be anxious to read this book, it has been directed primarily to the lay public. Technical terms and language have been avoided as much as is possible. I have no problem with that as over the years of my practice many patients have expressed their gratitude that I explained technical medical terms in everyday language. That also has been a frequent comment of readers during my 17 years of writing about the medical-dental problems in my "Nutritionally Speaking" column.

There is no question that in order to get technical subject matter across that many medical names of things have to be mentioned. I am concerned about the risk of turning people off as they could very well be the ones who most need to receive this information.

The secret of not being stumped by technical names is much like our handling the names of people we meet. Names like McCaffetory, Zubachelesky or Vibrestentz make us blink but we have no trouble conversing with these people after the introduction.

Now my name doesn't seem too difficult, still throughout my practice I found few who would address me by my last name because they didn't know how to pronounce it. A few caught on to saying Dr. George and that took hold and solved the problem.

So if you or some of your friends find the presence of those technical names a bit disconcerting, pass them by like you do those difficult monikers you run into when you meet someone. To test this out we had a number of non-science people read the galley proofs and although a number of them remarked about some of the difficult names of things (there are no substitutes for names you know) everyone of them understood what this book is all about.

I am pleased to tell you that before too long, and maybe even before this book is out, there will be another on this subject of root canal therapy. Dr. Hal Huggins has been repeating the Price research and has had some professional meetings about it with dentists.

He has been making great strides with both animal and human follow-up studies. Not being sure of just when the Huggins' research would be published I have been rushing ahead with exposing this cover-up because of my concern for the tremendous number out there who are suffering from focal infection disorders.

It is my hope the dental and medical professions will study what has been accomplished. To take a do nothing attitude and demand the usual push for more and more research will take many, many years, and cost millions of lives, not to mention billions of dollars of expense.

Certainly much additional research needs to be forthcoming. However, once you people out there read about the extent to which the Dr. Price studies were conducted, I believe your growing sophistication with health matters will result in your seeking whatever advise and help you need in order to determine what course of action will be best for you under your particular set of circumstances.

In pursuing the pages of this book what should be kept in mind is that every infected tooth, except those derived from injuries, started as a tiny cavity. Tooth decay is so common it is unfortunately considered a trivial matter. At the same time, dental care has become so efficient that our patients have come to believe dentists can solve whatever happens.

It is hoped the real objective and true purpose of this book will be achieved — that every reader will see to it that they have regular prophylaxis and oral examinations in order that any tooth decay that does takes place will be discovered at its very beginning. At that point there should be little danger of ever needing a root canal treatment.

The following three quotations seem an appropriate way to encourage your pursuit of the amazing discoveries of Dr. Weston Price that follow.

Life... is a predicament.

– Santayana

Things do not happen in this world.
They are brought about.

– W. Hays

To know truly is to know by causes.

– Bacon

ACKNOWLEDGEMENTS

In jotting down the name of the numerous people who have been of help to me in writing this exposé of the cover-up of the Dr.Weston Price root canal research, my effort came to an abrupt halt when I realized the number of names on the list hit 26 and was still not completed.

Among those whose counsel I sought for a wide variety of reasons were dentists, physicians, chiropractors, Ph.D.'s, relatives, friends and acquaintances. Each proved valuable and worthy of being acknowledged herein, but the length of the list made doing so impractical. I trust each of you will understand how much your help and words of wisdom are appreciated.

I will limit this list to those who, for the most part, were daily contributors in the task of writing this book. First there is my dear wife Eleanor, whose love and devotion made this undertaking possible; Sue Brydon for her always pleasant, cooperative ability in handling my many and varied typing requirements; Diane and Carl Rohkar for their computer expertise and ability to put all this into book form; Charlene Koonce for her enlightening and meticulous editing; Pat and Joe Connolly for their years of daily devotion and dedication to the Price Pottenger Nutrition Foundation; Hal Huggins for assuming the responsibility of bringing Dr. Price's work back to life and in repeating his research; my brother Doug, not only a fellow dentist but a co-member of the original 19 founders of the American Association of Endodontists; Dr. Jeffrey Bland for recognizing Dr. Price's work has not received the attention and acknowledgement it deserves and for his Forward for the book; Dr. Jerry Mittelman and his wife Bev for suggesting the "cover-up issue" would make for a better title and for his Forward; to Dr. Edwin Van Valey for so clearly recognizing the responsibilities of the dental profession in this matter and for writing an introduction to the book; and To Dr. Lendon Smith for his Commentary about immune system issues and of the importance of nutrition to the prevention of the need for root canal treatment.

To all of those named and to those un-named, I trust each of you will realize some inner pleasure in having played a part in bringing these important messages back to life. Please remember that each of you most certainly will have a beneficial effect on the health of millions of people.

INTRODUCTION

The book Nutrition and Physical Degeneration written by Dr. Weston Price in 1938 was a revelation to me many years ago, although the information that it contained was something that you always knew in your heart was correct. Dr. Weston Price was a man ahead of his time. His research was voluminous as well as his documentation. In this book, Dr. George Meinig has brought to light the Dr. Price work on endodontics which raises the question as to whether root canal therapy might endanger your life.

We, as endodontists, must look at Dr. Price's fascinating and thought provoking scientific papers as there is information in this research that some endodontists may be reluctant to accept. As members of one of the healing professions, we must search out the truth of his findings. As a practicing dentist, I am not a research scientist, but I implore those that are involved in research to look at this material, duplicate his tests and not dismiss his results out of hand. It is the obligation of those involved in endodontics to be aware of this material, and if it is true, and I think it is, to inform our colleagues and patients.

In 1919 my father, Dr. E.G. Van Valey (a founder of fourth President of the American Association of Endodontists) joined Dr. M.L. Rhein and in 1950 I joined the practice which continues to this day. My father lectured extensively and treated a large number of endodontic patients. Dr. Rhein started practice in the late 1880's, and early researcher in prevention and endodontics as well as a prolific writer who produced a film in 1917 showing procedures for performing root canal therapy much as it is done today. Dr. Rhein's father, who was a physician, disagreed with his son vehemently over treating patients with root canals arguing that he was doing more harm than good. Was his father right? Was Dr. Rhein right? Were they both right and wrong?

I believe it was Maury Massler who told us in a lecture one time to question what we learn as the truth in science, because half of what we know today is dead wrong — our main problem is to determine which half.

My awareness of the Price endodontic research about the possible harmful affects of root canal goes back several years. Since the saving of teeth has been a strong belief all my life, it has been difficult to accept Dr. Weston Price's research, but now I seriously wonder whether it was wise to treat all of those teeth. We all must keep open minds, however, and seek the truth.

The risk benefit ratio must be considered in contemplating a root canal procedure today, particularly if the patient's immune system is already compromised. The doctor and patient must come to a final decision taking into consideration this new-old information.

Edwin C. Van Valey, D.D.S., F.A.C.D, F.I.C.D.
Past President, American Association of Endodontists

COMMENTARY

We have found this to be outstanding. The information is critically important, and we can see your frustration that the world has not enthusiastically embraced these ideas.

We know of the work of Dr. Price, but had no idea of the extent of his research. The material you so carefully, fully, and clearly delineated comes at a time when the immune system is the key to just about everything that is alive.

You are right. This material needs to get to the people. It supplies one more reason why we must return to the diets of our ancestors. We cannot rely on toothbrushes and fluoride. The metabolism and the acid/base balance, and the calcium phosphorus ratio is the key to good health.

We would love to be more supportive of your work.

Lendon H. Smith, M.D.

CHAPTER 1

How a Rabbit Exposed the Problem...
Meet the World's Greatest Dentist

If you have ever had root canal treatment, and some twenty-four and one-half million people did last year, you are about to learn how that unfortunate necessity may have created greater side effects in your body system than you or your dentist could have anticipated.

What is to be revealed here is information of great importance to the life of every man, woman and child — and, what is more, it is new information even to those in the dental profession, for they too know very little about what I am about to disclose to you. It is information that, in spite of the numerous exhaustive scientific studies that have painstakenly been carried out, was — until now — shamefully buried.

For the most part, the evidence was driven underground and has remained there because of a general lack of interest by the dental profession during the early part of the century in the treatment of root canals. Secondly, and more importantly, there were serious disagreements within the dental and medical professions regarding the acceptance of the focal infection theory.

This theory stated that a person could have an infection someplace and that the bacteria involved could be transferred by way of the bloodstream to another gland or tissue and therein start a whole new infection. Dr. Price found that 95 percent of focal infections started in teeth and tonsils.

This is a story about how bacteria become trapped in teeth and tonsils and how important discoveries made about these bacteria and the diseases they cause have been hidden from the public and health professionals for over 70 years!

Unveiled is how these bacteria mutate, that is change form, multiply and — like the migration of cancer cells — metastasize, that is spread and infect the heart, kidneys, lungs, stomach, eyes, and countless other tissues.

This is a story about the world's greatest dental research specialist, Weston A. Price, D.D.S., M.S., F.A.C.D. and his focal infection research conducted under the auspices of the American Dental Association Research Institute and how he was silenced, causing a vast array of catastrophic, costly degenerative disease problems to engulf our people and nation.

This book will cover the remarkable extent and caliber of these investigations, how to reverse the destructive side effects of root canal therapy, and how people can become well again.

Come with me now and learn of Dr. Price's earthshaking discoveries. Here is a dedicated scientist whose work is recorded in 220 scientific articles and three major books that grace both dental and medical literature. Although millions have heard of his highly respected nine-year investigation into the natural cultural diets of 14 races of primitives living throughout the world and his research book, *Nutrition and Physical Degeneration*, his discoveries about the serious and dangerous side effects of root canal therapy are virtually unknown.

This compendium of that Dr. Price research will, at long last, disclose the extent and importance of his prodigious 25 years of most thorough studies about all aspects of root canal therapy.

More about why his monumental basic discoveries have not come to the attention of the dental profession or the public until now will be presented a little later in this book. Whether you presently have a root canal filled tooth or will need one in the future, let us get right into why this information is so important to you and people everywhere.

You don't have to be a dentist to understand this information. You will find it fascinating and inspiring, but at the same time quite frightening.

Dr. Price was imbued with the idea that dentists can't learn how to save teeth by taking them out. That in order to preserve teeth for a lifetime, each of us in the dental profession must accept our duty and responsibility to learn everything necessary to successfully combat the infections acquired by teeth. Even though in Dr. Price's time few dentists did root canal therapy, Dr. Price was as proficient in treating root canals for his patients as any dentist is today.

However, he had the sense that, even when such treatment appeared successful, teeth containing root canal fillings remained infected.

That thought kept preying on his mind, haunting him each time a patient consulted him for relief from some severe, debilitating disease for which the medical profession could find no answer. Then one day, while treating a woman who had been confined to wheelchair living for six years from severe arthritis, he recalled how bacterial cultures were taken from patients who were ill and then inoculated into animals in an effort to reproduce the disease and test the effectiveness of drugs on the disease.

With this thought in mind, he advised this arthritic patient, although her tooth looked fine, that she should have it extracted. He told her he was going to find out what it was about this root canal filled tooth that was responsible for her suffering.

All dentists know that sometimes arthritis and other illnesses clear up if bad teeth are extracted. However, in this case, all of her teeth appeared in satisfactory condition and the one containing this root canal filling showed no evidence or symptoms of infection. Besides, it looked normal on x-ray pictures.

Immediately after Dr. Price extracted the tooth and his patient was dismissed, he embedded the tooth under the skin of a rabbit. Lo and behold,

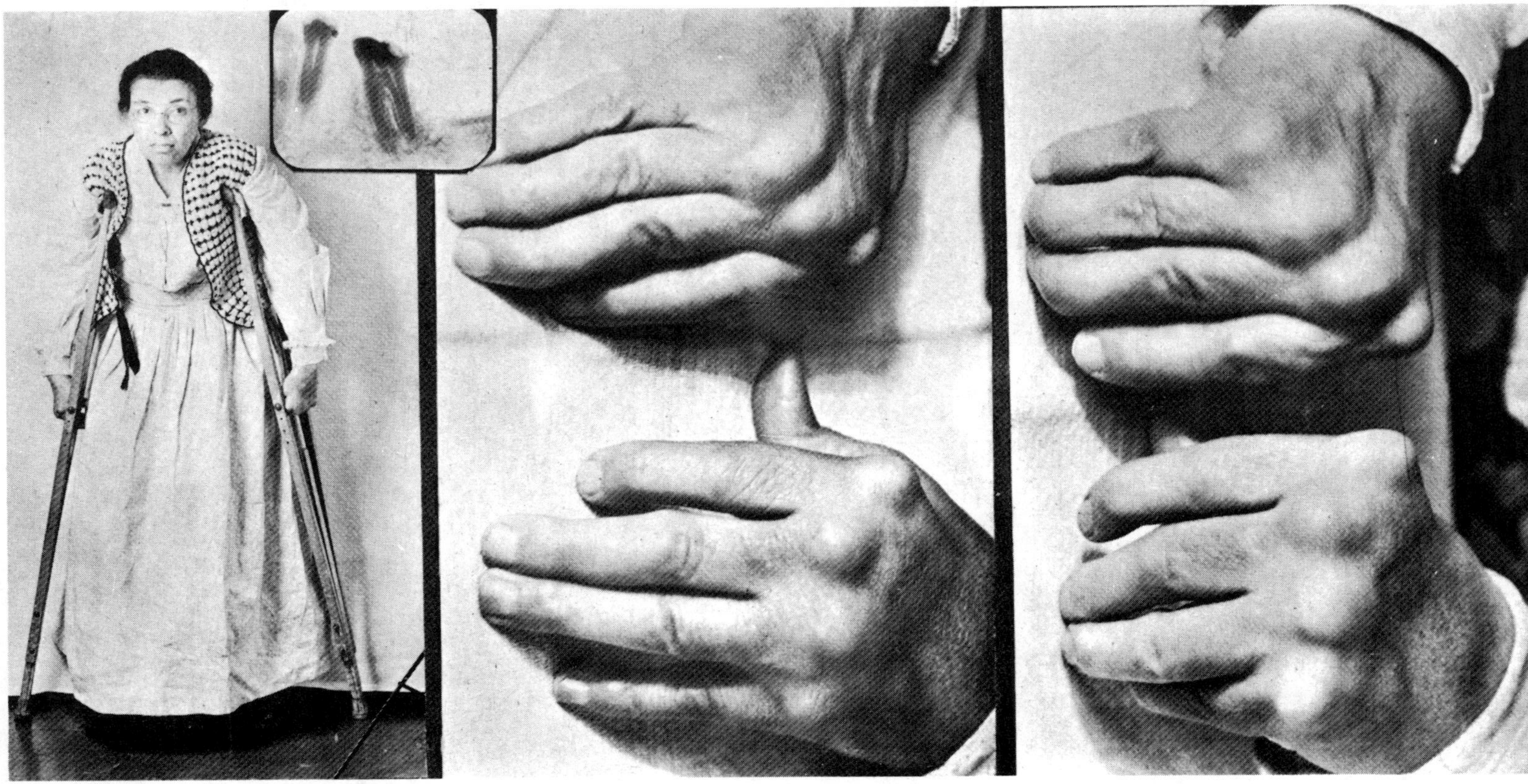

Chronic deforming polyarthritis. This woman was a bedridden cripple, completely helpless for six years. After extraction of infected tooth, she could walk about her house without even a cane and was able to do beautiful fancywork. Note condensing osteitis, not rarefying, about tooth. (Case No. 709)

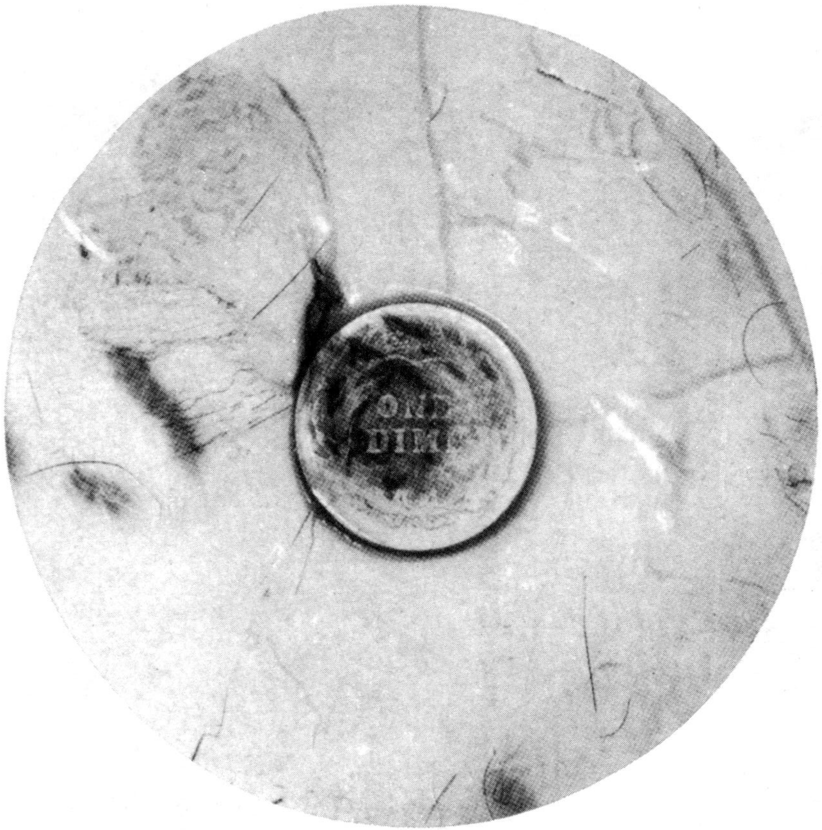

Appearance of a sterile coin two months after implantation beneath a rabbit's skin. No fibrous capsule formation or irritation — a slight etching of coin.

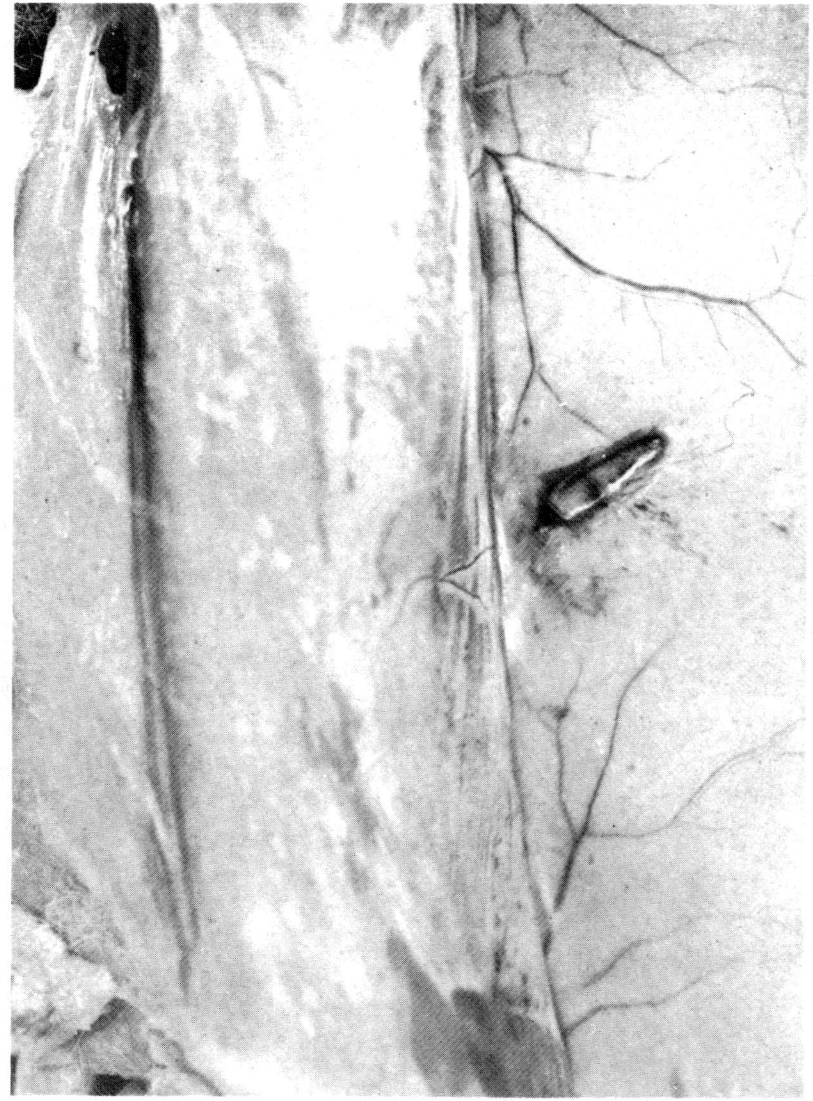

A sterile implanted tooth which produced practically no encapsulation nor any infection in the rabbit.

in two days the rabbit developed the same kind of crippling arthritis as the patient. What is more, in 10 days it died of the infection. (See accompanying picture of patient.)

You can readily see how such a discovery would excite a dental research specialist. What is more, the patient made a successful recovery after the tooth's removal! She could then walk without a cane and could even do fine needlework. That success led Dr. Price to advise other patients, afflicted with a wide variety of illnesses that were defying treatment, to have any root filled teeth removed.

Thereafter, whenever such situations occurred, he either embedded the whole tooth or small parts of the tooth under a rabbit's skin. Eventually he was able to obtain cultures of bacteria from within teeth and inject the cultured material into rabbits or other experimental animals. In almost every instance, the rabbits developed the disease of the patient or one similar to it. These infections proved so devastating that most animals died within three to 12 days.

If the patient had kidney trouble, the rabbit developed kidney involvement; if eye trouble, the rabbit's eyes failed. Heart trouble, rheumatism, stomach ulcers, bladder infections, ovarian diseases, phlebitis, osteomyelitis, whatever disease, the rabbit promptly became similarly infected and most — because the immune system of rabbits is poor — died within two weeks.

Dr. Price tested the theory further by implanting sound natural teeth under rabbits' skins, such as healthy teeth removed for orthodontic tooth straightening or those that were impacted and couldn't grow in properly. In addition, sterilized dimes and other coins were implanted and, in each instance, nothing detrimental happened to the rabbits.

These healthy teeth or coins lay dormant under the skin. Some developed a non-infected cystic sack about the objects and some exfoliated the foreign objects (pushed the coins or healthy teeth out of the skin by the action of the immune system), but these rabbits lived on in good health. None of them developed the illnesses that occurred to those that were inoculated with a bacterial infection from a root filled tooth.

Summary:

- Root canal fillings can cause serious side effects.

- Dental research specialist, Dr. Weston Price, after observing many patients with crippling degenerative diseases not responding to treatment, suspected infected root filled teeth to be the cause.

- Dr. Price devised a testing method that disclosed the presence of infection in a tooth that otherwise seemed to be healthy — that is, the implanting of the root filled tooth under the skin of a laboratory animal. He found, in almost every case, that when the root filled tooth of a patient with a degenerative disease was extracted and imbedded in an animal, that animal would develop the patient's disease.

- In the beginning, Dr. Price did not know just where the infection was hiding in the tooth, only that a patient's illness was rapidly transferred from their root filled tooth to laboratory animals in case after case.

- Dr. Price was later able to culture the bacteria in root filled teeth and trap their toxins, reproducing a disease in a rabbit by injecting the cultured material into the animal.

- Dr. Price discovered a wide variety of degenerative diseases to be transferable to rabbits, such as endocarditis and other heart diseases, kidney and bladder diseases, arthritis, rheumatism, mental diseases, lung problems, pregnancy complications, almost any degenerative problem — and after extraction of these teeth, a large percentage of patients recovered from their illnesses.

- When sound, uninfected natural teeth or other sterile objects were implanted in animals, no adverse health effects were experienced.

- Why this important research was forced underground, and has remained virtually unknown since its 1923 publication, will be covered in later chapters.

CHAPTER 2

Alarming Cover-up of Vital Root Canal Research Discovered

Anyone who starts to read this book is sure to wonder what in the world ever motivated a successful dentist and endodontist such as myself to state that *root canal treated teeth have side effects that cause many disorders!* Certainly my dental colleagues, particularly those who know me and are familiar with my background, are going to think I really flipped my lid.

How could a succesful dentist who was honored at the May 1993 five day 50th anniversary meeting of the American Association of Endodontists (root canal therapists) as being one of the 19 founding members of the organization ever come to publish a book of this critical nature?

On the other hand, who else but someone with this kind of background could appraise the serious research recently unearthed after 70 years of virtual oblivion?

Millions of people are ill and suffering from degenerative diseases for which the medical profession are at a loss regarding cause and treatment; and the degenerative disease problem continues to bankrupt our people and country. These two extremely alarming issues, and the light the root canal research sheds upon them, persuaded me to blow the whistle and alert the public to Price's substantial findings that could help them so tremendously.

My particular involvement as one of the 19 dentists who organized the Endodontic Association grew out of participation in the Dr. Edgar Coolidge Root Canal Study Group. At the time, Dr. Coolidge was the leading professor in the world about the subject of endodontia. He was not only my teacher of the subject but my mentor as well. Because so few dentists at the time were familiar with treating infected teeth, Dr. Coolidge and our group presented teaching clinics at dental meetings around the country.

Another circumstance contributing to my interest in this subject was my active participation for the past 20 years as a director of the Price Pottenger Nutrition Foundation. Yes, this foundation is the custodian of all the research memorabilia of the same Dr. Weston Price. The Foundation's main purpose has been to make his book, *Nutrition and Physical Degeneration*, available to the public and health professionals. His nutrition research project was initiated after the completion of 25 years of his root canal studies.

It was Dr. Price's belief that studying people and animals experiencing tooth decay and/or periodontal gum disease in order to determine why they developed these diseases was not the most effective approach. He felt that research emphasis should be on those individuals and animals that do not have these diseases, and then to determine what causes such diseases to henceforth evolve.

Price explored this theory with the same thoroughness and completeness that marked his other efforts. During a nine year period, he sought out primitive cultures living on native foods. During that time he visited and studied numerous tribes of 14 different races all over the globe.

Invariably, no matter what their native diets or where they lived, these people had excellent teeth, extremely low decay rates, very little — if any — crookedness of teeth, and no impacted teeth. He further noted that most were magnificent specimens of health, having few illnesses, physical or mental. The equivalent of jail was non-existent as these natives proved to have great mental and emotional stability.

On the other hand, when these same people came in contact with our civilization through the establishment of trading posts, rampant tooth decay took place and first generation children developed severe crookedness of teeth and many of the same diseases and malformations modern civilization exhibits, including cleft palates, hairlips, and club feet.

The items primitives received in trade were much the same everywhere: a few pieces of clothing, some trinkets, certain vegetable oils, jams and jellies, white flour, and sugar. No matter where in the world these primitives lived, 90% of the total items they received in trade consisted of white flour and sugar.

These two foods accounted for their severe degeneration and downfall. Clearly demonstrated was the fact that most diseases they developed after adopting these foods were not genetic but "environmental."

Price's 18,000 pictures, hundreds of slides, and numerous articles and books were the inspiration that started many nutritionists on their own pursuit of this subject.

As a director of the Price Pottenger Nutrition Foundation (P.P.N.F.), I was under the impression that I had seen and read most of Dr. Price's 220 articles, but somehow, although we had a copy of his two volumes on root canal therapy, they escaped the notice of all of us connected with P.P.N.F.

In 1992, the foundation's executive director, Pat Connally, received a call from Dr. Hal Huggins, a great admirer of Dr. Price's nutritional research. Dr. Huggins informed Mrs. Connally that a friend of his who had personally known Dr. Price called to say that, because of Hal's great interest in Price's nutrition work, he was sending two other Price books to him. This friend stated that "they contained information most important for the world to learn about" — that "the two volumes were interrelated and inseparable, needed to be pursued together, and that their message must not be allowed to die."

When the two books composed of 1174 pages and weighing nine pounds arrived, they were placed on Dr. Huggins' table. The first entitled, *Dental Infections Oral and Systemic*, is 703 pages long and the other, *Dental Infections and the Degenerative Diseases*, contains 471 pages. As this volume of information appeared to be a formidable undertaking, the books just sat for a long while on Dr. Huggins' table. After a couple of months of stealing glances at the books, curiosity got the best of Hal and he began reading the first one.

He excitedly told Pat that from the moment he picked the first book up he couldn't put the volumes down. He then briefed her about the extensiveness and greatness of the research, saying that the Foundation must get this unbelievably important work to the dental profession and the public.

Pat called me that evening with Dr. Huggins' story. Because of my vast experience in root canal therapy, it appeared that I should be the P.P.N.F. director to review the two books. As the foundation only had one original set, Pat had them copied and sent to me.

As soon as the copies arrived, I read the table of contents and couldn't believe the magnitude of the work Dr. Price had undertaken. I was terribly disturbed and shaken that I had never heard anything about his accomplishments. I began reading the books immediately and I, too, couldn't put them down. More and more, I became flabbergasted that our profession and the public has been cut off from learning about the basic and serious problems involved in this subject.

Since then, Dr. Huggins has set up a laboratory and is repeating Price's experiments. Because housing rabbits takes up so much laboratory space, he is using guinea pigs instead. So far his preliminary work indicates similar results to those found by Dr. Price. Dr. Huggins is beginning to present the Price story and his own research to the medical/dental professions; he has conducted two preliminary professional seminars about Price's root canal research and is planning others.

I was happy to learn that Dr. Huggins is presenting these discoveries to dentists and physicians. However, I am concerned that the subject's highly controversial nature will further delay this information getting from doctors to the public. It is worthwhile to keep in mind how many important advances in medicine have come about only after public pressure has been applied.

Considering the very large number of people who are ill with degenerative diseases that have proved insolvable by the medical profession, allowing the public to scrutinize root canal fillings as a possible cause of such diseases becomes urgent and further delay intolerable.

So, pressure built up for me to accept responsibility for alerting the public to the great implications of Dr. Price's research to current medical health issues. My being one of the original 19 charter members of the American Association of Endodontists, and having played an important role in the early development of that organization, would lend credibility to the book as would my experience managing the 20th Century Fox Studio dental office.

Then too, the 17 years experience of writing my "*Nutritionally Speaking*" column for the lay public in the Ojai Valley News newspaper and the publishing of my widely read book, *"NEW"TRITION — How to Achieve*

Optimum Health, also pointed to me as the logical person to carry this information to the public. Besides, who else was available with background and interest in this subject other than Drs. Huggins and Meinig?

But I kept asking myself, *"Is an ability to put technical language into readable form enough? Will this subject and its critically important messages only bring unrest to the public? Will my profession seize the information and utilize it, or will they be highly critical and disbelieving?"*

As you are now reading these pages, you can see that I bit the bullet and the book has become a reality.

I don't apologize for this long personal history, as it is necessary for you and my colleagues to know all of the background if you are going to fully digest and comprehend what is to follow. By now I'm sure you sense that this research took place a good many years ago. In fact, Dr. Price started investigating root canal problems in 1900 and the research continued past 1925. His two books on the subject were published in 1923.

Now I can hear many of you asking, *"What is this old 1920s stuff got that hasn't been superseded by all the great advances that have taken place in dentistry since that time?"* Well for your own sake, humor me a bit and stay with it. Root canal therapy was an important part of my practice. Still, until a year ago, I had never heard a word about Dr. Price's research on this subject and the basic nature of his discoveries.

Dentists have always been quick to grasp new methods and new ideas. Though this work was done long ago, it will be necessary for people to become acquainted with its revelations before they can judge whether what appears as old is actually very new. I am confident that my profession, after they look at the evidence, will see their own work in a different and broader light.

Oh, but I hear you say, as will my colleagues, *"Won't antibiotics now be able to solve the bacterial control problem?"* The answer to that is, "no" — I don't think they will, but let me briefly postpone explaining the reasons why I believe antibiotics will fail to work inside the tooth's intricate structure. Also, the fact is that — even if antibiotics could work inside the tooth — their use has not been standard treatment. Therefore any benefits, if they in fact exist, do not apply at this time to what is taking place.

In order for you to better appreciate the genius of Dr. Weston A. Price, let me divulge some notable information about him. The extent and depth of his efforts are difficult to comprehend as they were so extensive and thorough. Because of the number of investigations Price made, he was a most popular, sought after speaker for dental and medical meetings all over the country — and, in addition, he did numerous presentations to lay groups. Here is just a small sampling of his other research subjects that resulted in leading dental and medical journals publishing some 220 articles about his work:

The Movement of Positively Charged Particles
The Use of X-rays in Dentistry
Color Problems in Porcelain Work
Less Painful Dentistry
Laws of Governing Casting
Correction of Occlusion and Lengthening the Bite
Determination of Acidity and Alkalinity of Saliva
Special Researches in Physics
Correction of Facial Deformities
Newer Knowledge of Calcium Metabolism
Metallurgic Studies
Calcium and Phosphorus in Health and Disease
Control of Dental Caries
Butterfat, Vitamins and Seasonal Morbidity

Because of the extent of these many and varied endeavors, Price became known as a "Dental Research Specialist." This led, in 1915, to his receiving an appointment as the first Research Director of the National Dental Association — which, just a few years later, changed its name to the American Dental Association (A.D.A.).

Considering the size of the A.D.A. at that time, one might picture the Research Institute as a small organization. However, by then Price had more than 150 scientific articles published in dental and medical journals. This enabled him to attract support of the country's leading experts in the fields of medicine, dentistry, and business.

As President and Managing Director, Price had an organization of 60 members, of which there were nine trustees and five officers who ran the Research Institute for the A.D.A. He also secured an Advisory Board of 18 of the leading men of his time involved in the various sciences. Most of these men were famous for their own individual accomplishments. The names of a number of them, such as Dr. Charles Mayo, Dr. Frank Billings, Dr. Thomas Forsyth, Dr. Milton Rosenau, and Dr. Truman Brophy, will be familiar to many of you.

To understand the scope and impact of this and other projects by Price, it is imperative that you know what kind of help he had in formulating the various studies. Here is a list of the Advisory Board Members:

Advisory Board

Doctor Victor C. Vaughan, Dean of the Medical Department, University of Michigan; Ex-President, American Medical Association

Doctor Charles H. Mayo, President, Clinical Congress of Surgeons of North America; Surgeon, Mayo Institute, Rochester, MN

Doctor William H. Welch, Professor of Pathology, Johns Hopkins University, Baltimore, MD; President of the Board of Trustees, Rockefeller Institute

Mr. H.M. Hanna, Philanthropist, Cleveland, OH

Doctor Ludvig Hekteon, Professor and Head of the Department of Pathology, University of Chicago; Director, Memorial Institute for Infectious Diseases, Chicago, IL

Mr. Thomas Forsyth, President and Donor of the Forsyth Dental Infirmary for Children, Boston, MA

Doctor Frank Billings, Dean of the Faculty; Professor and Head of the Department of Medicine, University of Chicago, IL

Honorable Myron T. Herrick, Ex-Governor of Ohio; Ex-Ambassador to France; President, Society for Savings, Cleveland, OH

Doctor Milton J. Rosenau, Professor of Preventive Medicine and Hygiene, Harvard Medical School, Boston, MA

Professor Irving Fisher, Professor of Political Economy, Yale University, New Haven, CT

Doctor Robert S. Woodward, President, Carnegie Institute, Washington, D.C.

Doctor Edward C. Kirk, Dean, Thomas W. Evans' Museum and Dental Institute, Philadelphia, PA

Mr. Earl D. Babt, Attorney at Law, New York City, NY

Doctor Truman W. Brophy, Oral Surgeon; Dean, Chicago College of Dental Surgery, Chicago, IL

Doctor Louis W. Ladd, Assistant Professor of Clinical Microscopy, Medical Department, Western Reserve University, Cleveland, OH

Doctor Frank R. Lillie, Professor of Embryology; Chairman of the Department of Zoology, University of Chicago; Director of the Marine Biological Laboratory, Woods Hole, MA

Doctor Walter E. Garrey, Professor of Physiology and Physiological Chemistry, Washington University, St. Louis, MO

This Board, both personally and by way of their backgrounds, was able to provide Dr. Price with co-working scientists in the fields of bacteriology, pathology, rheumatology, immunology, chemistry, cardiology, surgery, and whatever other branches of medicine and dentistry that needed to become involved in the research.

Price had this to say about his co-workers:

> *In conducting the researches herewith reported, I have undertaken to secure the closest cooperation possible by engaging men for my staff whose exclusive attention has thereby been concentrated on the particular phase for which they were engaged. There has, therefore, been the closest possible cooperation without the possibility of distraction or conflicting purpose; and I am profoundly indebted to these collaborators, who have been many, during these two and one-half decades, in working on these problems.*
>
> *No work on this subject can be presented at this time, if at any time in the future, without recognizing in a very important way the exceptional pioneer work that has been done by Dr. E.C. Rosenow, first while working in Chicago at the Presbyterian Hospital in association with Dr. Frank Billings, and latterly in the Mayo Institute at Rochester, Minnesota. Probably to Dr. Billings more than to any other American internist is due the credit for the early recognition of the importance of streptococcal focal infections in systemic involvements, for his work practically paralleled that of Sir William Hunter in England.*
>
> *I wish to express my deep indebtedness to all these pioneers in this field; and if my work shall have removed some of the confusions which have been largely responsible for the lack of appreciation of, and opposition*

to, the efforts of these great pioneers, I should be doubly glad because of my esteem for their courage in the midst of the bitterest of opposition, and also for the larger helpfulness that may come to humanity by a more universal medical and dental appreciation of this need. There could not possibly be a stronger tribute to the sincerity of these men than that they should so persistently follow the line of their conviction in the midst of the unprecedented antagonism, for theirs was the vision of a great new truth."

Not only did Dr. Price direct the endeavors of these illustrious scientists, but he spent half of each day's time at the Research Institute.

Dr. Price refused to take any pay for his endeavors and, in fact, donated much of the equipment used in the Institute's laboratories.

The studies involved thousands of patients, an average use of 500 rabbits each year, and a representative group of other laboratory animals as well.

The following two pages are the title pages of the two Price books. They are worth reading as they summarize the importance of this earth-shaking research.

DENTAL INFECTIONS
ORAL AND SYSTEMIC

(VOLUME I)

BEING A CONTRIBUTION TO THE PATHOLOGY OF DENTAL INFECTIONS
FOCAL INFECTIONS, AND THE DEGENERATIVE DISEASES

By

WESTON A. PRICE, D. D. S., M. S., F. A. C. D.

Specialist in Dental Research and the Diagnosis, Prognosis, and Treatment of Dental Infections.
Chairman Research Section of The American Dental Association, 1914 to present.
Organizer of The Research Commission of The American Dental
Association. Organizer of The Research Institute of
The American Dental Association
(Discontinued)

THIS IS THE EXPERIMENTAL BASIS FOR VOLUME II
"DENTAL INFECTIONS AND THE DEGENERATIVE DISEASES"

VOLUME I PRESENTS

RESEARCHES ON FUNDAMENTALS OF ORAL AND SYSTEMIC
EXPRESSIONS OF DENTAL INFECTIONS

VOLUME II PRESENTS

RESEARCHES ON CLINICAL EXPRESSIONS
OF DENTAL INFECTIONS

From the Author's Private Research Laboratories
8926 Euclid Avenue, Cleveland, Ohio

THE PENTON PUBLISHING COMPANY
Scientific Publishers
PENTON BUILDING CLEVELAND, OHIO

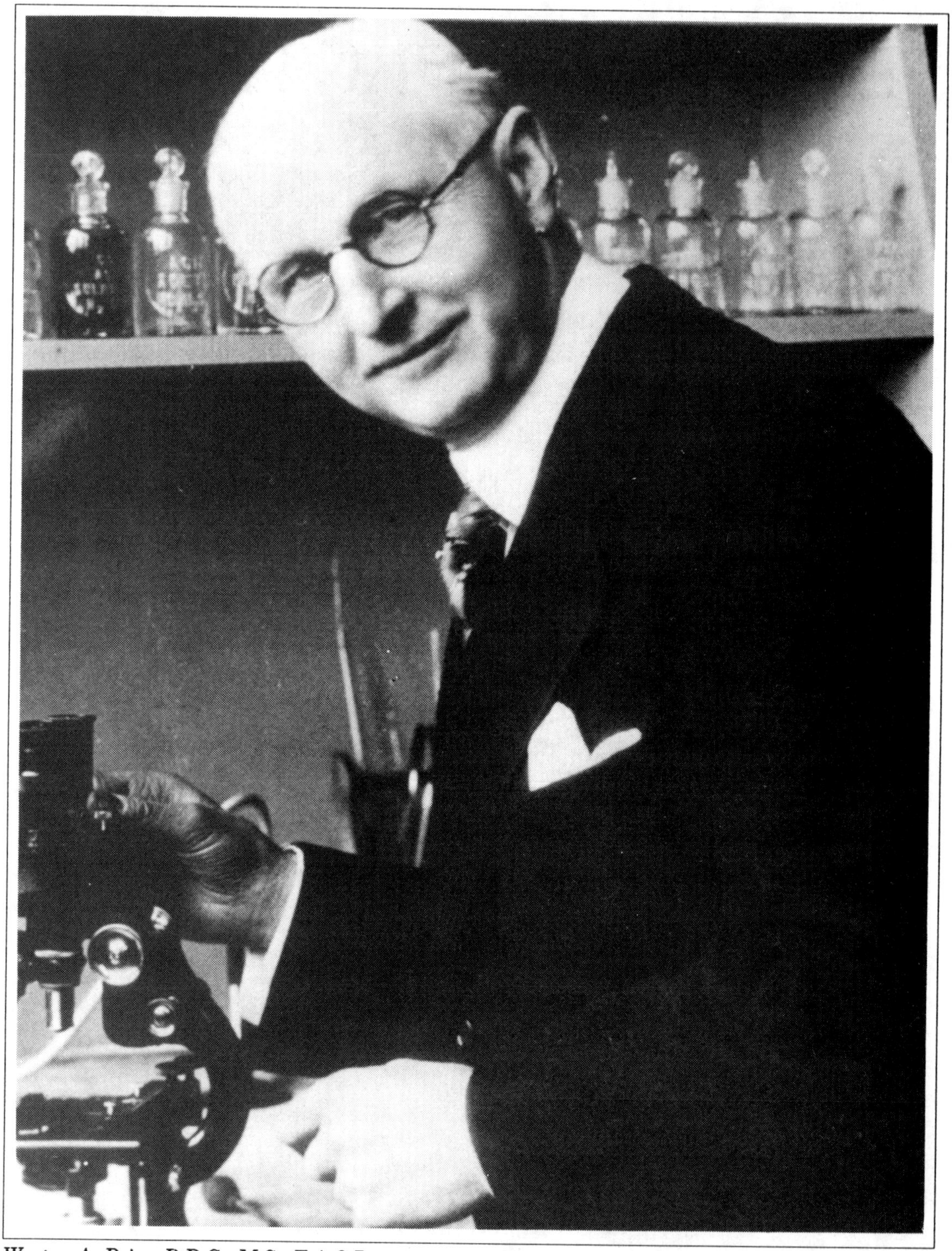

Weston A. Price, D.D.S., M.S., F.A.C.D.

DENTAL INFECTIONS
AND THE
DEGENERATIVE DISEASES

(VOLUME II)

BEING A CONTRIBUTION TO THE PATHOLOGY OF FUNCTIONAL AND DEGENERATIVE ORGAN AND TISSUE LESIONS

By

WESTON A. PRICE, D. D. S., M. S., F. A. C. D.

Specialist in Dental Research and the Diagnosis, Prognosis, and Treatment of Dental Infections.
Chairman Research Section of The American Dental Association, 1914 to present.
Organizer of The Research Commission of The American Dental Association. Organizer of The Research Institute of The American Dental Association
(Discontinued)

THIS IS THE CLINICAL ASPECT OF VOLUME I
"DENTAL INFECTIONS, ORAL AND SYSTEMIC"

VOLUME I PRESENTS
RESEARCHES ON FUNDAMENTALS OF ORAL AND SYSTEMIC EXPRESSIONS OF DENTAL INFECTIONS

VOLUME II PRESENTS
RESEARCHES ON CLINICAL EXPRESSIONS OF DENTAL INFECTIONS

From the Author's Private Research Laboratories
8926 Euclid Avenue, Cleveland, Ohio

THE PENTON PUBLISHING COMPANY
Scientific Publishers
PENTON BUILDING CLEVELAND, OHIO

Summary:

- Background history of how this book came into being covered the author's activities as a member of the Dr. Edgar Coolidge Root Canal Study Group, clinic lecturer to dentists encouraging treatment of infected teeth, and organizer — one of 19 — of the American Association of Endodontists (root canal therapists).

- Presented was how it came to pass that Dr. Hal Huggins was given two books written by Dr. Weston Price along with the responsibility of keeping the basic research contained therein alive.

- Dr. Huggins, seeing the importance of the Price discoveries, accepted the responsibility and is repeating the research experiments. He alerted the Price Pottenger Nutrition Foundation (P.P.N.F.) to the degenerative disease implications.

- Because of the author's background and experience, P.P.N.F. encouraged his review of the Price root canal research data.

- In order for readers to accept such reporting, it is essential for them to know the background qualifications of the original researcher (Dr. Weston Price) and secondly, that of the person reporting these investigations (Dr. George Meinig).

- The Dr. Weston Price qualifications:
  * He earned a Masters of Science degree in his native Canada, Doctor of Dental Surgery from the University of Michigan, and a Fellowship in the American College of Dentists.
  * Because of his extensive research efforts, he became known as a Dental Research Specialist — and those efforts led to his being referred to as the "world's greatest dentist."
  * His dental investigations resulted in the publication of 220 scientific articles and three long books.
  * These activities led to the American Dental Association appointing him President and Managing Director of its 60 person Research Institute.
  * His Advisory Board of 18 consisted of the leading doctors of his day, the names of whom some of you will recognize: Dr. Charles Mayo, head of the Mayo Clinic; Dr. Frank Billings who coined the term "Focal Infection"; Dr. Milton Rosenau, Preventive Medicine professor, Harvard University; Dr. Truman Brophy, Dean of the Chicago College of Dental Surgery, etc. (The names of the full board are listed.)

* Dr. Price's other accomplishments, awards and citations are too extensive to mention here but are covered in the chapter.

* After reviewing the two Price books for the Board of Directors of the Price Pottenger Foundation, Dr. Meinig was encouraged to put the technical data into book form for the lay public.

- The qualifications the Foundation found pertinent in their choice of Dr. Meinig were:
  * Doctor of Dental Surgery degree from the Chicago College of Dental Surgery
  * Forty-seven years of practice including three years in the air force during World War II
  * Clinic lecture experience about root canal therapy
  * Active participation as one of the 19 founding charter members of the American Association of Endodontists (root canal therapists)
  * Broad background practice in most branches of dentistry
  * Management of the 20th Century Fox Studio dental office
  * 20 years service as Director of the Price Pottenger Nutritional Foundation
  * Became a fellow in the American College of Dentists (F.A.C.D.)
  * 17 years experience writing the *"Nutritionally Speaking"* column in the Ojai Valley News newspaper
  * Authorship of the widely read book, *"New"trition — How to Achieve Optimum Health*
  * Lectures on a variety of dental subjects in numbers of states and four foreign countries
  * Status as one of the first holistic dentists
  * Practice of root canal therapy

- Also presented in this chapter was a direct Price quotation regarding the support his research endeavors received from leading doctors of the time. All branches of medicine and dentistry were represented on his research team, including bacteriology, pathology, rheumatology, immunology, chemistry, cardiology, and surgery.

- It should also be noted that Price devoted half his time to conducting the studies at the A.D.A. Research Institute, taking no pay for his efforts and donating much of the equipment used.

CHAPTER 3

The Bacteria and Other Microorganisms That are Involved in Dental Infections

A crucial factor in root canal infections is the role of bacteria. Price and the Research Institute's bacteriologists and other key workers isolated the same streptococcus, staphyloccus, and spirochete families of organisms from the teeth and mouth as investigators find today. Although any one of these organisms could be causative of the oral infections people suffer, they found that over 90 percent of the time the bacteria involved were of the streptococcus species.

The chart below, reprinted from Dr. Price's book, lists the technical names of the bacteria and how often they caused infections of the teeth and mouth. The bar graph pictorially depicts the frequency that each type of germ was involved.

RELATIVE PREVALENCE OF DIFFERENT STRAINS

*Type of Streptococcus	%	Graphic Expressions
Fecalis	65½	
Ignavius	1½	
Salivarius	1½	
Infrequens	9	
Mitis	7½	
Non-Hemolyticus I	3	
Non-Hemolyticus III	3	
Hemolyticus I	3	
Subacidus	1½	
Pyogenes	4½	

The chart below, also from Dr. Price's book, again lists the types of bacteria found in the teeth and mouth, and lists the specific diseases each caused.

Type of Lesion in Patient	S. Ignavius	S. Salivarius	S. Infrequens	S. Mitis	S. Non-Hemolyticus I	S. Non-Hemolyticus III	S. Hemolyticus I	S. Subacidus	S. Pyogenes	S. Fecalis	Percentage S. Fecalis	Ratio of Chance
Rheumatism			2		1	1				**7**	11	**7.1**
Heart										**2**	3	**1.3**
Nerves		1	3	4	2	1	2		3	**21**	33	**24.05**
Lassitude			2	1						**11**	17	**9.1**
Internal Organs		1	1	1						**8**	13	**7.1**
Special Tissues	1		3	1		3				**7**	11	**9 7**
No Lesions								1		**7**	11	**5.2**

With the preceding factors in mind, we can now look into the reasons why these organisms find teeth and their surrounding tissues such lovely places to live. Bacteria regard the inside of teeth as attractive a home as we do a Frank Lloyd Wright dwelling in a beautiful setting. The following picture of a tooth will help you to see why organisms find teeth and gums such a perfect hideaway.

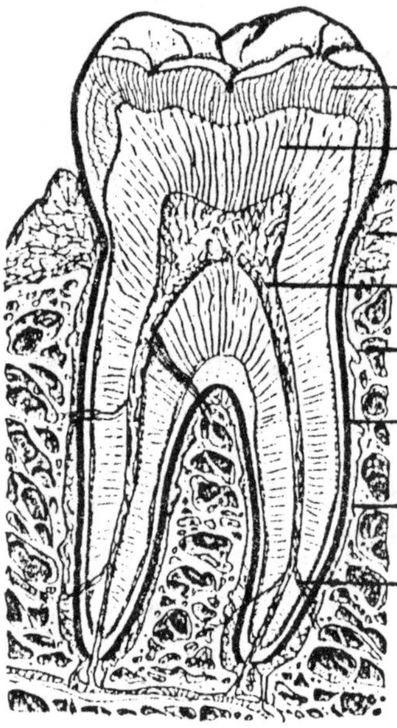

You will note that the crown of the tooth is covered by a hard, shell-like covering of enamel. The majority of the tooth substance is called dentin. It isn't as hard as enamel. The dentin of the root of the tooth is covered by cementum. It is harder than dentin but not as tough as enamel. The reason for you to know these details about tooth structure will become clear as we proceed with the description of what happens to rabbits and other animals.

The following paragraph is quoted directly from one of Price's books:

> *"In the physical structure of the tooth with the dentin connected chiefly, if not solely, with the pulp, and the cementum connected chiefly, if not solely, with the periodontal membrane, we are dealing with two structures, each sufficiently porous to give habitation to millions of organisms. We have shown elsewhere that the dentinal tubuli of a single-rooted tooth comprise enclosed canals totaling approximately three miles of length, but each of these two structures is formed on a practically continuous homogeneous base, the dentin and cementum being backed up to each other."*

It will surprise you to learn that when a dentist cuts only the enamel of a tooth, no pain is involved unless the tooth becomes overheated by a fast moving drill or diamond stone. Once the dentin just under the enamel is contacted, however, most people experience discomfort. While it was previously believed that there were no nerve fibers in dentin, electron microscope studies of the dentin tubules now show they do contain very fine nerve fibers. (Frank, 1966; Arwill, 1967; Brännström, 1981)

The dentin isn't as hard as enamel because it is composed of tiny hollow tubules, so small they can only be seen through a microscope. These dentin tubules have a number of characteristics and functions that are very important to our understanding the process of tooth infection.

The tubules contain a fluid and this fluid carries nutrients and other matter needed by teeth to keep them healthy. To accomplish its tasks, the fluid movement that originates in the pulp on the inside of the tooth flows to the enamel and even through the enamel. Yes, the hard enamel substance is porous enough to permit such movement. It is this fluid that nourishes all parts of teeth and is responsible for giving them life.

By now numbers of scientists have documented this interesting phenomenon and have demonstrated that the fluid flow in the dentin tubules from the pulp outward is actually reversed when a person eats sugar. In more recent years, Dr. Ralph R. Steinman, Professor Emeritus from the Loma Linda University Dental School, found in studies of rats that the flow reversed when he injected glucose (sugar) under the skin of their abdomen.

He also introduced sugar directly into their stomachs through the use of a stomach tube and had the same result. This, contrary to popular belief, showed that sugar doesn't have to touch teeth at all for its presence to result in a severe amount of tooth decay. These investigations clearly demonstrate that the reversal of fluid flow in the dentin tubules could be created by detrimental nutritional changes that, in turn, would be responsible for severe systemic changes to the bodies of humans and animals.

When tooth decay penetrates the enamel of the tooth's crown, the bacteria that are always present in the mouth and are actively involved in the decay process enter into the dentin tubules and progress along inside of them. They are also part of the carious process that keeps eating away more and more of the tooth substance.

Once the decay gets close to the pulp, the bacteria travel the full length of the inside of the tooth via the tooth's arteries and at the same time enter into the dentin tubules all along the border of the pulp.

Now, when the tooth develops pain from an infection and a root canal treatment is performed and the filling placed, these bacteria become sealed in the tubules. Incidentally, medications dentists use to sterilize the root canal have more or less been successful, but Price proved they had no effect against the bacteria found in dentin tubules.

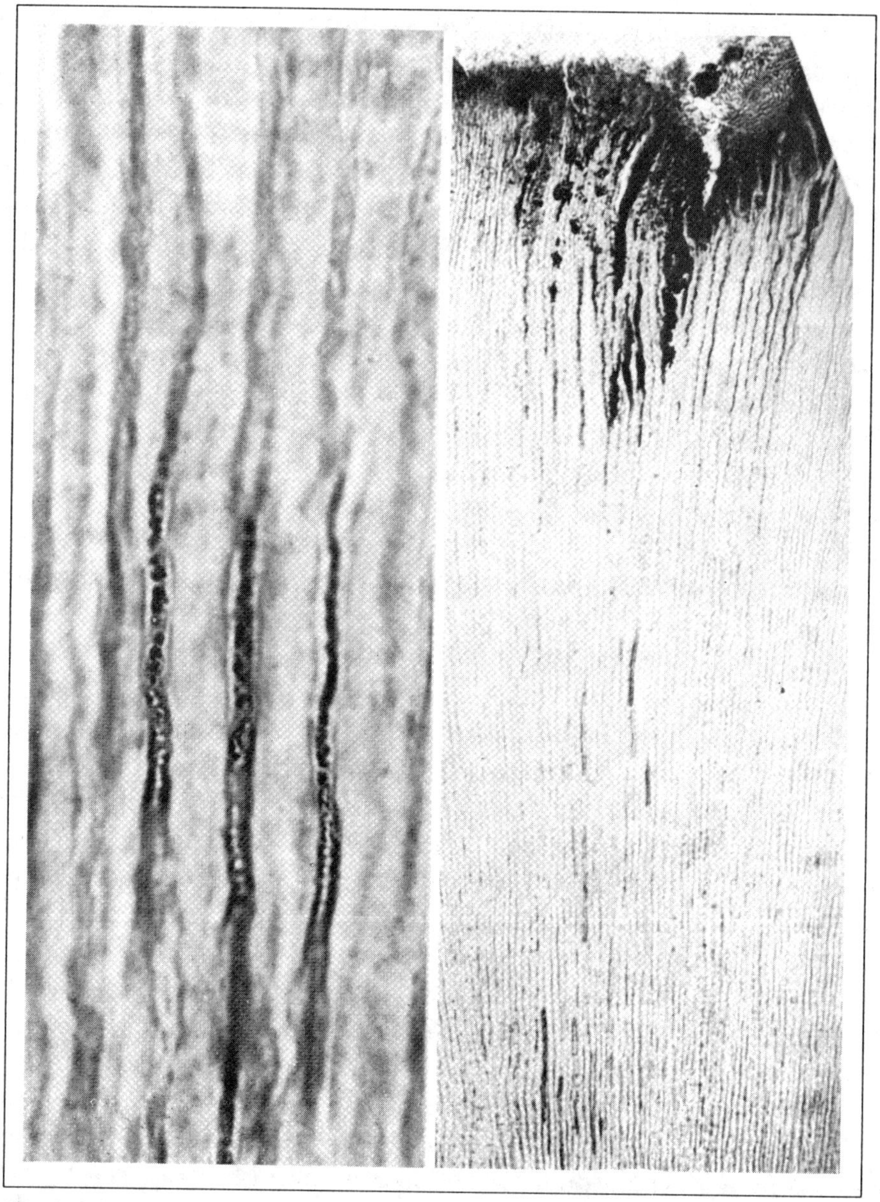

The low power magnification picture on the right shows tooth decay just starting on the enamel surface and how far it has penetrated inwardly.

The picture on the left shows an enlarged magnification view of bacteria present in dentin tubules.

Most bacteria involved in tooth infections were believed to be aerobic types; that is, they need oxygen to survive. More recent studies indicate that bacteria found in infected teeth for the most part are anaerobic, that is they do not need oxygen to live. However, this discovery — by way of the two studies of Ake Möller and Lars Fabricus in 1981 in Sweden — involved monkeys, not humans. It would be easy to assume that the aerobic bacteria in the dentin tubules would die off when the root canal filling is placed as its presence would seal off the tubules, thereby preventing their obtaining air.

But they don't die. They are very hardy beasts, and are polymorphic; that is, they mutate — change form. They become smaller in size and number and they now can thrive in the absence of oxygen. At the same time they become more virulent and their toxins much more toxic.

It might be of interest that the Wall Street Journal, on the morning of my typing this page, reported that one year ago a small group of scientists had met and exchanged data on the first drugs discovered by major pharmaceutical companies to arrest the AIDS virus. Their euphoria was blown just six months later when they found the AIDS virus wasn't being controlled but was mutating, and in its new form the infection was able to begin all over again.

The article went on to say that because of the organisms' ability to adjust and change, scientists now feel it may be a long time, if ever, before there is a cure for AIDS. Isn't it interesting that so long ago Dr. Price found that bacteria trapped inside of teeth were doing the very same thing!

Getting back to the mutating streptococci germs or other bacteria housing themselves in dentin tubules, the obvious question is: "So what, how can they escape?"

If you go back to the picture of the tooth, you will see that not only is there a main root canal, there are also some smaller, lateral canals. These actually allow bacteria in the vicinity of these accessory canals to escape through the cementum and into the alveolar process (the bone network that holds a tooth in the mouth). That bone, of course, has a blood supply that nourishes it and those blood vessels can transport the bacteria they pick up to all parts of the body, thereby allowing the organisms to select any organ, gland or tissue they feel would make a good second home.

The cementum itself won't allow the bacteria through its dense substance, except through accessory canals. However, the cementum is not able to stop the toxins of the bacteria from seeping through its structure.

In another investigation, Dr. Price explored this possibility using extracted teeth. He cemented small steel tubes into the root canal from the tooth's root end. He then hooked these up to a device that would pump water into the root canal under pressure. He found that when a dye was introduced, the colored water not only traveled through the dentin tubules but seeped through the entire structure of the cementum: the roots' outer, seemingly impervious, protective covering.

In addition to these ways for bacteria to escape into the bloodstream, bacteria can also leak out from around the root canal filling material. Dentists diligently try to pack the root canal filling material so that it doesn't permit bacteria trapped in the dentin to leak through the root filling material and out through the root canal opening at the end of the root, but tests by Dr. Price and others have shown that leaks occur.

You should now be able to visualize how bacteria and their toxins escape from teeth and travel the bloodstream to tissues near and far away. Sooner or later they find a suitable gland or organ and set up housekeeping anew. This is one of the ways that organs and other tissues become infected and diseased.

This process was formerly called focal infection. Many physicians and dentists in Price's time strongly disagreed that teeth, tonsils or other infected areas surrounding teeth could be responsible for an infection being transferred to another part of the body. From the evidence of the Price research you can readily see, by the dramatic recovery of most patients upon the extraction of their infected root filled teeth, and by what happened to rabbits when infected teeth were inserted under their skin, just how these illnesses occur and why they frequently do so.

But what about those people who have had root filled teeth for years and have had no problems? Dr. Price found these patients to have remarkably good immune systems that were able to control the bacteria and keep them at bay, thereby allowing the person to function in reasonably good health.

However, Dr. Price found that when such people had an accident, caught the flu bug, had a death in the family, or suffered some other severe stress situation, the overtaxing of their immune system could, at that time, allow the development of rheumatism, arthritis, a heart problem, or any one of a number of other diseases. Anything that overly stresses the immune system can allow bacteria trapped in the teeth to multiply and travel to cause illness in some other part of the body. Dr. Price referred to this as a failure of the "body defense system." Today we call it a weakness in the "immune system."

Changes that were found to occur in the blood from dental infection are a low white blood cell count (leukopenia), a deficiency of red blood cells (erythropenia), an increase in the number of white blood cells formed in lymph tissues (lymphocytosis), and a tendency to hemorrhaging (hemophilia). In addition, changes in the body content of ionic calcium takes place and pathologic quantities of calcium accumulate in the blood. The alkaline reserve is lowered and acidosis occurs. There is an increase in blood sugar, uric acid, nitrogen retention, and products of imperfect oxidation develop.

Each of these areas of change that occur because of the presence of dental infection was thoroughly investigated by Dr. Price. The area that produced the most confusion and required extensive research time was that of the role of calcium. Every cell of the body is dependent on the presence of ionic calcium. It is used in teeth and bones, in the movement of muscles, the rhythmic action of the heart and intestines, and is indispensable for the coagulation of blood at the time of cuts, injuries, surgeries, etc. More about the significance of calcium will appear from time to time as the report of Dr. Price's research continues.

Summary:

- The Price team of bacteriologists isolated the same families of streptococcus, staphylococcus and spirochetes found in root canals reported today.

- 90 percent of bacteria in teeth that produced patients' diseases in animals were streptococcus and 65½ percent of the time they were of the fecalis family. Current bacteriologists today find Dr. Price's discoveries were accurate.

- Dentin, that makes up the majority of a tooth's structure, is the key to understanding the chronic infections present inside of teeth.

- The hard, solid appearing dentin is actually made up of tiny tubules that carry a fluid that transports nutrients from the tooth's blood supply to all parts of the tooth.

- The tubules are so small that one needs a microscope to see them. The number of tubules in a single rooted front tooth would form a chain three miles long if they were attached together end to end .

- Dr. Ralph Steinman, Professor Emeritus at the Loma Linda Universtiy Dental School has shown that the fluid movement in dentin tubules flows from the pulp, inside of the tooth, outward and through the enamel and cementum — and that this movement is reversed when sugar is eaten, even when injected into laboratory rats or introduced by way of a stomach tube.

- A picture in one of Dr. Price's books shows the presence of bacteria inside of dentin tubules as soon as the first sign of tooth decay took place in that tooth.

- In all my schooling and 47 years of dental practice, I never saw a picture of bacteria in dentin tubules. Last year I came across such a picture in one of Dr. Price's two books published in 1923.

- When decay causes a tooth to become infected and abscessed, dentists are usually quite successful in cleaning out the root canal and disinfecting it. In most cases large areas of bone destroyed by the infection heal and new bone grows to replace it.

- In spite of this seeming success of root canal therapy, Price discovered that bacteria that caused the infection penetrated most of the dentin tubules and were not killed during the root canal therapy.

- Dr. Price found these bacteria to be polymorphic — that is, they mutated, became smaller in size, thrived in the absence of oxygen, and became more virulent and their toxins more toxic.

- How bacteria trapped in dentin tubules escaped into the body's general circulation of blood was a key question that caused much debate. Dentists even in Price's time were aware that infection could be present in a tooth's lateral accessory canals (see picture of tooth) and could become a source of infection elsewhere in the body.

- The hard, shell-like covering of the dentin — cementum — proved able to prevent the passage of *bacteria* from the roots of teeth. However, tests devised by Dr. Price showed that cementum did permit the *toxins* created by bacteria to pass through it.

- Bacteria could escape from the tooth through miniscule spaces or porosity of the root canal filling material. Here again, Dr. Price devised ways to test various root canal filling materials and packing methods for leakage. *None* proved successful in preventing the escape of organisms. All leaked into the bloodstream surrounding the tooth.

- What about those people who have had root canal fillings for years and have remained in good health? Dr. Price found these individuals represented about 30 percent of those treated and they had excellent immune systems that were able to control the germs that were present.

- Nevertheless, when these same healthy people suffered a severe accident, a case of the flu, lost their job, or suffered some other unusually heavy stress that overtaxed their immune system, they could develop a degenerative disease problem because their defense mechanisms had become overwhelmed.

CHAPTER 4

Root Canal Disinfectants Prove Inadequate

In observing the transfer of so many illnesses of patients to rabbits, Dr. Price realized that the dental profession's supposition that the medications used to sterilize infected teeth were adequate and proficient must be considered fallacious. During the 75 years preceding his research many formulas were considered efficient in destroying the bacteria that infect teeth.

The criteria that dentists used then in determining the success of root canal treatment is the same today: the absence of discomfort and pain, and x-ray evidence that the abscessed areas, granulomas and cysts that were visible previous to treatment had healed completely. Although dentists believe such success is indisputable considering the evidence, Dr. Price put the soundness of such conclusions to the test by carrying out a number of experiments.

Dentists today will be surprised to learn that Dr. Price and his colleagues were making cultures from inside teeth to determine the presence of bacteria as far back as 1915 and perhaps earlier. As a dental school student, my contemporaries and I had to perform such a process but were under the impression that this was a new procedure. Few dentists, even today, use such a test to verify whether they have successfully sterilized a root canal.

During treatment, dentists place a Johnson & Johnson absorbent point saturated with a sterilizing medication in the patient's tooth for a few days in order to kill the bacteria that are causing the infection. The dentist then removes the dressing and runs a dry, sterile absorbent point into the canal, withdraws it, and places it in a test tube containing a culture medium that easily encourages the growing of bacteria.

When no growth occurs on the J&J point, the dentist concludes that the bacteria causing the infection have been destroyed and the root canal filling is placed. When bacteria growth is still present, sterilizing treatment medication is repeated until no bacterial growth is evident. Dentists have been taught that negative culture tests are proof of successful sterilization.

Price made tests of over a hundred different medicaments, including different strengths of each. With only eight of the medications was he able to obtain negative culture responses at the end of 24 hours, and very few were negative after being in the root canal for 48 hours. Testing for longer periods showed that negative test results were impossible to obtain since medication loses its disinfecting power.

In case you have any question about Dr. Price's ability to adequately treat root canal infections, the following x-ray picture of two central incisors he treated around 1910 indicate that they were as good as any treated today.

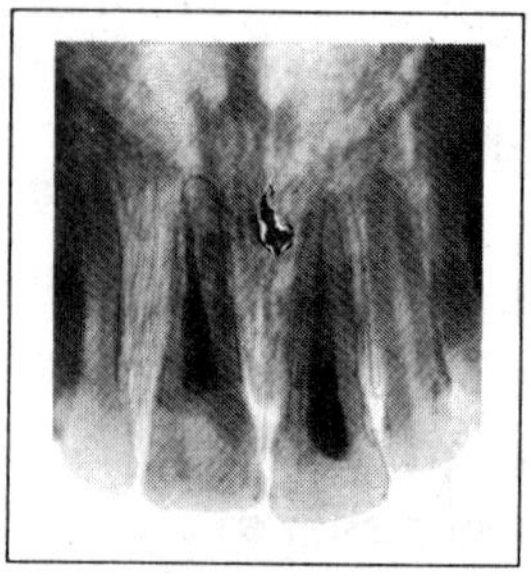

Two root canals treated by Dr. Price in the early 1900s.

Getting back to his study of medicaments, the two most efficient ones were found to be silver nitrate and formalin. However, both proved objectionable: silver nitrate because it turned the tooth black and formalin because it was very irritating to patients and destructive to the tooth's surrounding tissues. The medication that showed the most universal promise was chloramin-T (Chlorozene), a medicament our professor, Dr. Coolidge, taught us to use as students and one I used in my practice.

In another very revealing series of tests, the root canals of extracted teeth that had been removed because of abscessing were cleaned and sterilized. Using aseptic techniques, the teeth were sectioned and both the dentin and cementum cultured to see if they had been effectively sterilized. In each instance, both the dentin and cementum of all teeth tested showed them still to be infected. The only exception was when concentrated formalin was used. It showed sterility during 93 percent of the tests. However, when formalin is used in the mouth, it produces so much pain that it cannot be used.

In a case similar to that of the arthritic patient shown in Chapter Two, Dr. Price made a small incision at the gum line before the extraction, and with a curette removed some bone at the neck of the tooth. Not only did tests on the roots and cementum prove that they were loaded with bacteria, but the bone right next to the tooth's root was profusely infected as well.

These experimental tests demonstrated to Dr. Price that the belief previously held by himself and his profession — that infected teeth could be readily and effectively sterilized — was incorrect and that teeth could only be sterilized in a small percentage of cases and with great difficulty, or by using overly strong medicaments.

He concluded that he thought it possible that the dentin in young people could be sterilized to its junction with the root's protective cementum covering, but that it was improbable that the cementum itself could ever be sterilized by medicaments placed in the pulp chamber and root canals.

Now, most of you will be confident that with the use of modern antibiotics sterilization can be achieved. The chance of this, however, appears to be remote as antibiotics would need to penetrate all the miles of dentin tubules that make up dentin to kill all the bacteria that reside in them. Just how difficult the sterilization of teeth has proven to be will be covered in later chapters. The physical make-up of dentin and cementum is more complicated than has been realized and taught.

Contrary to my conclusions to date about the possible use of antibiotics to sterilize teeth and kill all bacteria, Dr. Price noted that the future development of medicaments such as antibiotics might bring more success and that this possibility, when such medicaments are developed, must be thoroughly investigated.

Summary:

- The criteria dentists use to determine whether their treatment of a root canal infection has been successful, namely the absence of discomfort and pain; x-ray evidence that abscessed areas, granulomas and cysts have completely filled in with new bone; and trust that the medicaments used in producing these results completely irradicated bacteria, proved inadequate when such teeth were subjected to further testing by Dr. Price and his group.

- Testing for the presence of bacteria in root canals, after the use of disinfectants which appeared to have controlled the infections, proved that the organisms had not been irradicated.

- Dr. Price, in making cultures after the use of over 100 different medicaments, including different strengths of each, found only eight that had negative responses after 24 hours and only two after 48 hours of incubation; longer periods were found to be ineffective as medicaments lost their disinfecting power.

- The two most efficient medicaments proved to be objectionable — silver nitrate because it turned teeth black and formalin because it was very irritating and painful to patients and destructive to surrounding tissues.

- Though culturing to determine whether bacteria had been killed was formerly taught and practiced, I know of no dentists using such a testing procedure today.

- Dr. Price in another series of tests took extracted infected teeth (much easier to do aseptically outside of the mouth), treated them and found that when these teeth were sectioned their dentin and cementum were still infected.

- In still another investigation, Dr. Price made biopsy sections at and below the gum line and found bacteria present not only in the roots of the teeth and their protective cementum but also in the first millimeter or two of adjacent bone. The importance of this factor in causing cavitations in bone after extractions will be discussed in a later chapter.

- Price noted that future developments might bring forth medicaments that are more successful. You will all be thinking that antibiotics are certainly the answer. However, there is great question as to whether antibiotics will be able to effectively penetrate the dentin tubules, cementum and adjacent bone sufficiently well to irradicate these bacteria.

- Testing of new medicaments, and current efforts such as new laser treatment methods, are — of course — necessary and were anticipated by Dr. Price.

- All of these root canal side effect problems should not deter the profession from continuing to explore new methods of how to save teeth. While we can't learn how to save teeth by extracting them, fortunately Dr. Price has shown us ways to test procedures to prove infection has been irradicated in those teeth we have saved that were infected.

CHAPTER 5

The Astonishing Blood Changes Produced by Dental Infections Emaciation and Weight Loss

In undertaking these studies, Dr. Price felt it would be of help to learn of any research disclosing what happens to a patient's blood when a dental infection is present. Sadly, he could find little in dental or medical literature, nor were his learned advisors able to furnish any information as to the impact of dental infections on human blood.

In order to better understand what happens to patients and rabbits when infected by oral pathologic bacteria, Dr. Price jumped right in and studied that problem with his usual thoroughness.

He made blood studies of patients suffering from dental infections and found that the number of polymorphonuclear leukocytes (a form of white blood cells that have nuclei with a variety of forms) were less than the normal average. At the same time, he noted that the number of small lymphocytes (white blood cells formed in lymph tissue) increased. He also noted that these changes returned to normal levels when the dental infection was removed.

In studying rabbits after infected teeth were implanted under their skin, he found that blood changes occurred in these animals in the same way. That is, polymorphonuclear white blood cells decreased 33 percent in number from their normal, and lymphocytes increased by 58 percent. Slight changes were produced in the number of mature red cells (erythrocytes): in some cases these decreased, in others they increased.

The amounts of hemoglobin in the rabbits changed very little. In some it stayed the same and in others the amount present reduced slightly. Hemoglobin is the red protein found inside of red blood cells that is responsible for the red color of blood.

A common occurrence is lymphocytosis. This is an increase in the number of lymphocytes: a form of white blood cell formed in lymphoid tissue throughout the body. They increase during the presence of infection in order to help dispose of the bacteria that are present.

Hemophilia, a marked spontaneous tendency to hemorrhage, was frequently a problem in rabbits inoculated with human tooth infections. Another was glycemia: high amounts of glucose in the blood. In addition, alkaline body reserves lowered, creating acidosis. There was increased uric acid and nitrogen retention.

In some instances, a higher level of ionic calcium was found in the rabbit's blood, but in most cases the level of ionic calcium became lower than normal.

This resulted in 15 to 20 different pathological conditions. These conditions will be discussed in the chapter on how our bodies and lives depend on free ionic calcium.

All rabbits that had inoculations of infected material involved in dental infection, or had infected teeth implanted under their skin, lost weight. The more severe the infection, the greater the weight loss.

Dr. Price noted that patients suffering from rheumatic diseases were prone to the withering away of their tissues. The emaciation could range from 10 to 25 percent in ordinary cases and 35 to 40 percent in extreme ones. He reported that one woman patient who had a normal weight of 130 dropped to 72 pounds. Upon removal of her dental infections, her weight quickly climbed from 72 pounds to 111. A culture taken from one of her infected teeth was inoculated into a rabbit. In four days time this rabbit had a weight loss from 1381 to 1105 grams (20 percent).

In another report, a male patient stated that he felt fairly well, that nothing was particularly wrong with him except that he was progressively losing weight. In this case there were no root canal treated teeth in his mouth, but he did have moderate to severe periodontal disease with several pyorrhea pockets so deep and full of pus that they had to be extracted. One of these teeth was crushed, washed and centrifuged. The clear solution that resulted was inoculated into a rabbit that in 16 days had a loss of weight from 1430 grams to 843 grams, a 41 percent drop. In counting the number of organisms under a microscope, it was calculated that the amount inoculated into this rabbit was only about one millionth of a gram — a very small amount.

To test the matter still further, they passed the washings of crushed teeth through a Berkefeld Filter that was designed to filter out all bacteria. When the remaining solution was injected into other rabbits, they still developed a marked loss of weight and had an average length of life afterwards of only five days. In these cases, because bacteria had been eliminated, the cause for their wasting away had to be the escape of remaining toxins from bacteria through the roots of the teeth.

In a group of 667 successive rabbit inoculations, some with cultures, some with filtrates of cultures, and many with filtered washings from crushed teeth, all were found to be bacteria free. Of these, $33^1/_3$ percent (or 220) lost 10 to 30 percent of their weight in a few days or weeks immediately following the injections; 8.7 percent lost 30 to 50 percent in weight; 13.6 percent gained from 10 to 30 percent; while 3.6 percent gained from 30 to 50 percent.

Inasmuch as all of the rabbits were maintained on the same diet throughout these tests, these changes in their blood and weight, whether up or down, must be considered diagnostic symptoms of the presence of dental infections, either from action of the bacteria or their toxins.

Summary:

- Dr. Price supposed that dentists would know if any changes took place in a patient's blood when a dental infection was present but he found no reports in scientific literature on that subject. This led him to do exhaustive blood studies of patients and animals to determine the side effects of root canal infections.

- Thousands of blood tests on patients and animals infected by root filled teeth showed:
  * Lymphocytes (white blood cells) increased in humans and increased 58 percent in rabbits.
  * Polymorphonuclear leukocytes, a form of white blood cells, decreased in humans and in animals to 33 percent less than normal.
  * Hemoglobin changed very little, either up or down.
  * Hemophilia, a tendency to hemorrhage, occured frequently in rabbits.
  * Increased amounts of sugar were found in the blood.
  * In some rabbits, higher amounts of ionic calcium were found; but in most rabbits, calcium was lower — resulting in 15 to 20 different pathologic conditions.
  * There was increased uric acid and nitrogen retention.
  * Alkaline reserves decreased, resulting in acidosis.
  * Some patients and all animals lost weight.

- Patients suffering rheumatic diseases often experienced a withering away of their tissues.

- Patients with pyorrhea pockets loaded with pus suffered severe weight loss, as did animals inoculated with diluted solutions of the crushed pyorrhetic teeth that had all the bacteria filtered out. This demonstrated dramatically that the toxins of the bacteria, rather than bacteria itself, caused the weight loss and death of the animals.

- Should you think this may have been an accidental or occasional occurrence, this study involved 667 rabbit inoculations.

CHAPTER 6

How the Different Root End Infections Affect the Body

When a dentist tells a patient they have an abscessed tooth, the term is rather loosely used to indicate that an infection is present. In the main, there are three quite different types of infections that take place at the root ends of teeth. They are: condensing osteitis, granulomas, and cysts.

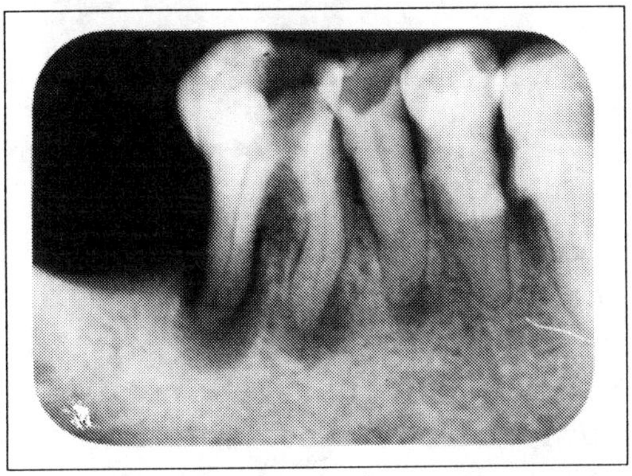

Root end infection from deep caries.

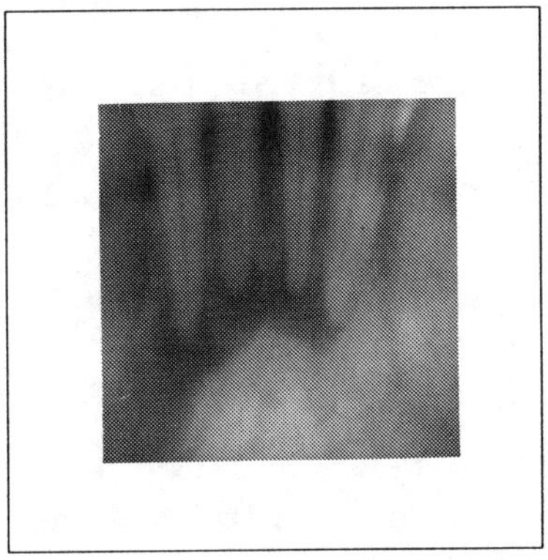

Root end infections from auto accident.

The granuloma is the most common. It shows up as an area at the end of the root about the size of a pea. Its size can be smaller or larger, depending on how soon the patient experienced a toothache and/or an x-ray picture was taken that disclosed its presence. The outer limits of the infected area have a skin-like sac that confines the spread of the infection but doesn't stop it from growing. The area that is seen on an x-ray picture is actually a hole in the alveolar bone that has been eaten away by organisms and/or their toxins.

Condensing osteitis cases have two main characteristics. In one there is a rather liberal amount of bone destroyed at the end of the root and the bone just adjacent to the infected area becomes very dense and hard.

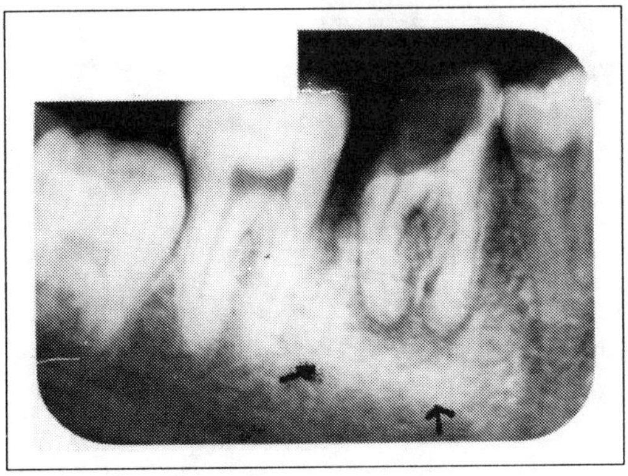

Condensing osteitis.

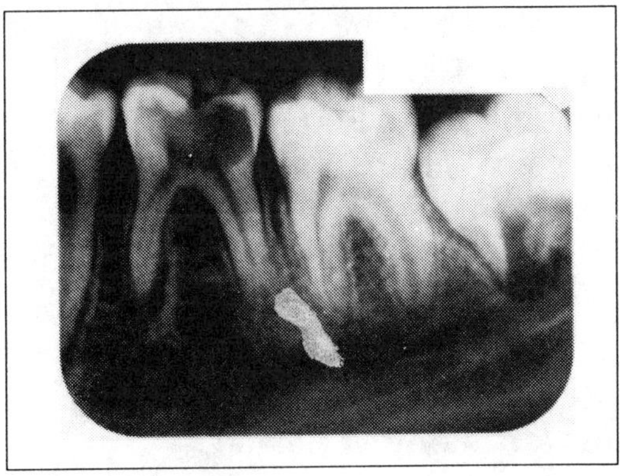

Condensing osteitis.

The other type of condensing osteitis shows very little, if any, loss of bone at the root end but it too has a dense, hard area that shows up clearly on x-ray pictures. In this case, the hard area is close to the end of the tooth's root.

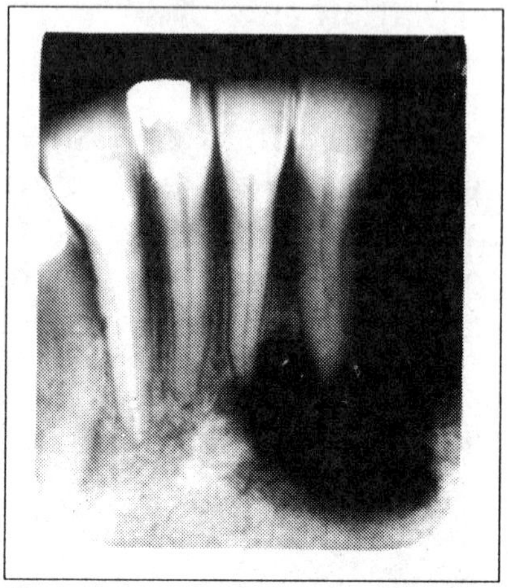

Cyst.

Cysts are a different kind of infection and are often not discovered until they become quite large. Their outer skin-like sac is of different tissue than that of the granuloma, and all of the cyst must be removed surgically when extracting the tooth or it tends to remain and keep growing.

Some infected teeth also have a fistula, a small tube draining pus from the infected area into the mouth or through the skin to an area on the face somewhat in proximity to the infected tooth.

Dentists at the time of Dr. Price's research, as well as those practicing today, generally consider that the larger the area of infection seen on an x-ray picture, and particularly those that have fistulas, the greater the severity of the disease. A careful study of 1400 patients showed this assumption to be false and that the type of lesion is a predictor of the kind of systemic body involvement that can take place.

For example, those showing condensed bone and very little change at the root end of the tooth proved to be the more serious infections. People with this condition were frequently found to be prone to a degenerative group of diseases.

On the other hand, those with large areas of alveolar bone loss and/or fistulas were generally found in patients in good condition with little or no systemic involvement. This has led to some confusion in the medical and dental professions, as the large numbers of patients presenting in outpatient clinics of hospitals — often those with low incomes — usually have more abundant infections than are found in any other group. On the whole, these people were found to have quantities of pus flowing from any number of broken down teeth, but Dr. Price found that most of these patients did not exhibit signs and symptoms of systemic illnesses. He demonstrated that the physical change about the root of the tooth was not a measure of its infection but was primarily related to the patient's body defense capability.

Today we refer to the body's defense capability as the ability of the person's immune system. If a person's defense mechanism is strong, Price speculated that there is localized spread of the infected area without the spread of organisms to other parts of the body — until the infection is present for a prolonged period.

Dr. Price reasoned that when the patient's defense is poor, the body tries to wall off the infection by surrounding the area with dense bone, and it is this dense bone that slows the growth of granulomas and stops fistula formation and its function of quickly carrying off pus. In these cases, the organisms' main means of escape to other parts of the body is via the bloodstream.

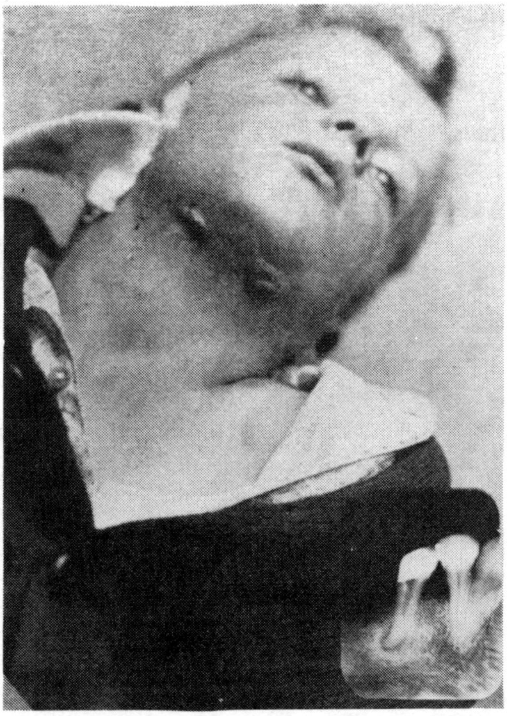

Fistulas draining pus from infected second bicuspid shown on x-ray insert.

The poorer the defense capability of a patient, the more probable that the bacteria will reestablish themselves in a new tissue or organ. Teeth in these cases tend to become more tender and painful than those that appear more seriously involved.

These results and conclusions encouraged Dr. Price to examine the bacterial content of granulomas, fistulas, and other areas of infection. Surprisingly, he found but few bacteria in such cases. Not only was the defense ability of these patients very good but the content of the pus flowing from fistulas consisted almost wholly of neutralized products. The few bacteria present were engulfed by white cells and, even more surprising, such areas were often sterile. The flow of pus carrying off the infectious material was actually serving to clear up and get rid of the waste products of the infection. *All of this is just the opposite of what appears to be happening and what dentists have been taught is taking place.*

In tests of granulomas and their contents, these were found to have a few more bacteria than those with a fistula, but for the most part the organisms present appeared to be well controlled by the white blood cells. Furthermore, it was discovered that the granuloma sac was a defensive membrane capable of destroying organisms and toxins, thereby aiding the immune system and helping to prevent systemic reactions.

In the condensing osteitis cases of patients with poor defense, the tissue at the end of the tooth's root was incapable of controlling the organisms and, in fact, seemed to aid in the transport of organisms into the blood and then to various organs, glands, and other tissues.

Cysts are quite a different form of infection that occur at the root ends of teeth. Although in their early stages they look like granulomas. Usually they cause no apparent symptoms or pain until they are quite large. They may be the result of tooth infections and are quite often caused by injuries. They can exist entirely in bone or soft tissues. They are well outlined by a skin-like membrane and contain a watery fluid that sometimes has a cheese-like consistency.

Dr. Price reported a number of cases of cysts that caused systemic involvements. One was a patient of age 76 who suffered a very severe central nervous system disturbance and had blood pressure so low that he almost died on several occasions. His physician diagnosed his condition as a heart block. After the removal of a tooth and its root end cyst, the patient's symptoms entirely disappeared. He could then walk for miles as rapidly as a 30 year old.

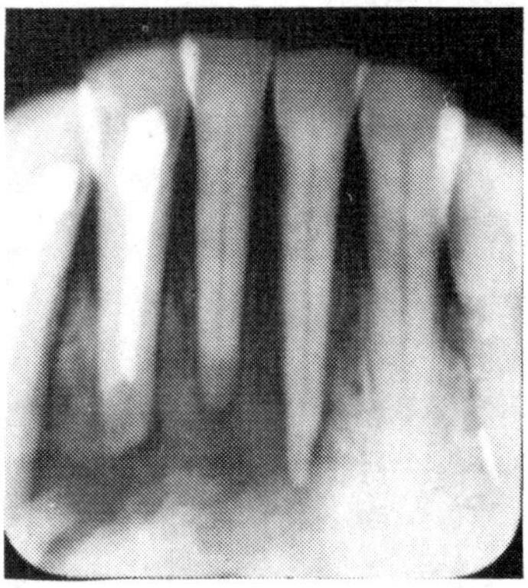

Cancer showing bone loss around three teeth.

Just the opposite occurred to another patient whose blood pressure ran above 220 but returned to normal after his tooth and cyst were removed.

Then there was the man who had an enormous cyst about an impacted wisdom tooth. This patient had colitis that resulted in bowel movements every 30 minutes. Rabbits inoculated with the contents of the cyst each developed diarrhea in about forty minutes and several developed severe spastic colitis.

One other case history involved a boy of 15 having a pulse of 160 and marked shortness of breath. When an infected cuspid baby tooth and a large cyst that was found below it were removed, the boy's heart condition subsided, allowing his pulse rate to drop in a few hours to 80.

The picture above of three lower front teeth involved with cancer shows a very infrequent manifestation of this serious disease. The infection in this case, though it resembles the granuloma or cyst infections commonly seen about teeth, is quite different in that the borders of the area are very irregular and unlike those of the typical dental infection. This cancer did not arise from the teeth but was a metastasis transfer from the original cancer located in the floor of the mouth. Most oral cancers are found to be caused by the use of tobacco, either from its use in smoking or from snuff placed in the cheek.

Dr. Price felt that not only the organisms but also the toxic substances produced by them had a great deal to do with the conditions of such patients. Although cysts are not as common as other dental infections, they prove just as devastating to many patients. Dr. Price felt that those who experienced cysts but few systemic disturbances had better body defense mechanisms.

Dentists reading this chapter may have trouble believing the observations of Price. In several places throughout his reports Dr. Price stated quite frankly that he fully expected the validity of his observations to be questioned. He added that although he felt confident of his conclusions, future research could prove that other factors are involved than what appeared to be indicated by his research procedures. His foremost concern was in finding truth.

It must be pointed out that to some extent the dental health of the American people was far worse during the first three decades of this century than it is today. Most people in previous times only went to the dentist after they had suffered for days and days with severe toothaches and swollen jaws. The majority of our citizens are availing themselves of more regular and better dental care than what was available in Dr. Price's time. There were a few exceptional dentists such as Dr. Price whose dentistry was comparable with that of today, but this was not the general case.

Bob Hope's weekly broadcasts for the Pepsodent Toothpaste Company following World War II sent more people into dental offices with his, "You will wonder where the yellow went, when you brush your teeth with Pepsodent!" and "See your dentist twice a year!" than anything we dentists were able to accomplish over decades with our altruistic prevention programs.

The point is that the huge number of severely diseased oral infection problems that Price had to deal with would make some of the percentages and statistics he details to be out of proportion to that prevailing today. This in no way detracts from the basic nature and soundness of his discoveries.

Summary:

- There are three main kinds of root end tooth infections, but in most instances they are simply referred to as "abscessed teeth."

- The three main root end tooth infections are called granulomas, cysts, and condensing osteitis.

- Granulomas and cysts, though they appear to be quite similar, have distinctly different characteristics.

- Fistulas are channels that carry pus from the infection area to the outside of the face or mouth. They help the body get rid of excessive amounts of pus.

- Condensing osteitis is rarely mentioned as a root end infection process but Price found its presense to be accompanied by some very specific infection related reactions.

- Dr. Price made bacteriologic examinations of these different dental infection areas. To his surprise he found, for the most part, that no matter how large an involved area or how much pus was flowing, comparatively few bacteria were present. He interpreted this to mean that the body's white blood cells and other defense mechanisms had good control of the infection process that was present.

- Furthermore, in such cases he found the patients to be in relatively good overall health and that they did not exhibit the expected signs and symptoms of systemic illness.

- Dr. Price reasoned that the large areas of bone destruction and pus about these infected areas were not a measure of the severity of the infection, as so commonly believed, but were in actuality expressing the goodness of the involved patient's immune defense capability.

- He further found that though the organisms spread locally, they did not spread to other parts of the body until the infection had persisted for a prolonged period of time.

- Condensing osteitis cases proved to be quite different. This condition exhibits a very dense area of bone, sometimes with very little loss of bone at the tooth's root end.

- Patient histories and in-depth studies revealed that people exhibiting condensing osteitis suffered more serious consequences from their infections. Price surmised that in such a case the patient's defense system was poor and that the body was trying to wall off the infected area with dense bone in order to contain its effects.

- However, the tissue at the root end was incapable of controlling the bacterial growth in these cases and consequently some bacteria escaped through the bloodstream and set up diseases in other areas.

- Price also noted that the teeth of such patients became more tender and painful than those cases that *appeared* to be more seriously involved.

- These observations by Price are so diametrically opposite of the average dentist's view and comprehension of what is occurring that many will have difficulty accepting these findings, in spite of the fact that they were derived from studies of 1400 patients.

- Numbers of case history examples were mentioned in this chapter to lend insight into these different infections and their effects. Included was a picture of cancer of the lower jaw below the roots of three lower front teeth that would appear to be a typical dental infection.

- Such examples were shown to emphasize that there are other dental disease conditions than those mentioned but they represent a much smaller proportion of cases and are not indicative of the average person's experience.

- Periodontal and other gum infections are in a different category. They will be discussed later in Chapter 10.

CHAPTER 7

Also Present — Spirochetes, Amoeba and Other Mouth Organisms

In Chapter Three it was pointed out that of the large variety of organisms inhabiting the mouths of people it was the streptococcus family that, through thousands of bacteriologic tests, Dr. Price found to be mainly involved in infections of the teeth and gums. He discovered that out of the 10 varieties of streps involved in mouth infections, the "fecalis" streptococcus was represented in $65^1/_2$ percent of the cases tested. Though streptococcus predominated, it was often accompanied by fellow organisms, such as those of the staphylococcus, spirochete, or protozoa families.

One of these species of microscopic travelers in our bloodstream would find some organ or tissue of the body an ideal place to set up housekeeping. Their sexual proclivity, by which they can divide and multiply, allows them to dominate the world in which they reside and makes for some severe illness situations.

The Price studies weren't able to disclose the extent to which *spirochete* forms enter the human body and are involved in dental infections, but his group's research led them to believe that these organisms do so more often than was, or is, realized.

Though systemic involvement in laboratory animals from spirochetes was a rare occurrence, a huge tumor-like mass on a rabbit's knee and a large abscess in the thigh of another rabbit — both of which were produced by introduction of an almost pure culture of spirochetes — are easily seen in the root canal microscope slide pictures of Dr. Price's study. Incidentally, the infections in these rabbits occurred after inoculations of organisms taken from a pyorrhea pus pocket of a patient suffering from an unusual type of neuritis.

The influence of spirochete infections upon the health of people can be both severe and rapid. Thorough medical scrutiny failed to disclose why a man lost 18 pounds in weight in three weeks. Oral examination, however, disclosed a chronic case of Vincent's infection, today often called acute necrotizing ulcerative gingivitis. With prompt dental treatment, the patient gained back 10 pounds in two weeks.

This infection is commonly called trench mouth because so many American soldiers in the trenches of France during World War I developed the disease. I can testify that the rates of cases were also high in the air force bases in this country during World War II.

Its cause is known to result from the joint action of a spindle-shaped germ tapered at both ends, the fusiform baccilli and a spirochete. Both of these organisms are generally present in most mouths, but become pathogenic when a person becomes debilitated, nutritionally compromised, or badly neglects the care of his or her mouth. It is now known that diet and nutrition play a big role in its inception. The B complex vitamins, niacinamide, vitamin C, and minerals have an active place both in treatment and prevention.

Current research reports in both the *New England Journal of Medicine*, August 22, 1991, and *Lancet*, November 9, 1991, disclosed that the spirochetes involved in trench mouth are from the treponema pallidum family and, although these spirochetes are cousins to those which cause syphilis, there is no reason to conclude that any form of gum disease is related to that sexual disease. When the syphilis infection is present, its particular spirochetes do show up in the mouth but effects are entirely different than those of Vincent's infection.

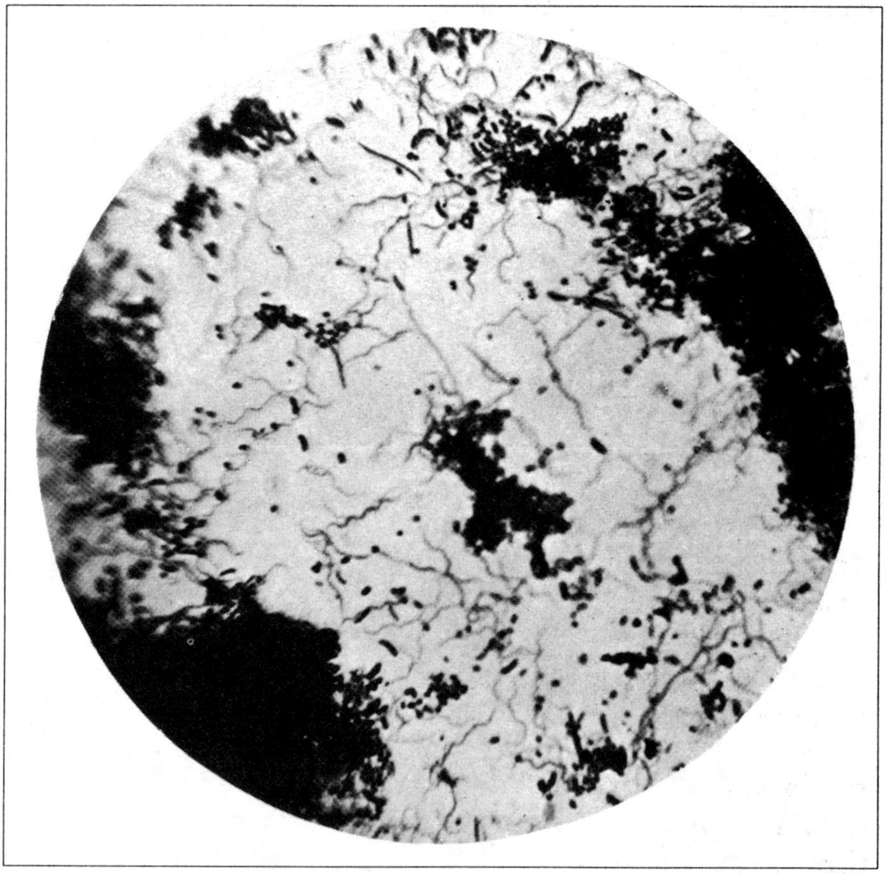

Culture of spirochetes from trench mouth, which caused patient to lose 18 pounds in three weeks. With local treatment, he gained 10 pounds in two weeks.

In understanding this dichotomy it would be well to know that 10 treponema spirochete species have been detected in periodontal gum infections and the exact one or combination has not been fully ascertained. In fact, some investigators feel these organisms may simply be opportunists that enjoy traveling with the fusiform bacillus.

During World War II, when I was stationed at the army air force base in El Paso, Texas, there were many cases of trench mouth and I was placed in charge of treating these patients. The local favorite treatment then was chromic acid. Response to this treatment was slow and the disease kept returning. It was just at that time that penicillin was released for use to the air corp dental clinics.

There were no reports as to the use of penicillin for Vincent's infection but it was well-known to be effective against most streptococcus and spirochete bacteria. We had no idea how best to use it, but after consultation with the pharmacy department, a mouthwash was prepared.

The soldiers were instructed to take one mouthful every hour, holding it there and swishing it around vigorously before spitting it out. Well, the results were spectacular and unbelievable; in only one day there was very noticeable improvement. The foul breath was gone, bleeding lessened considerably, and patients could eat most foods without discomfort. In three days, all signs of infection were gone. We had so many soldiers on the base with a mouthwash bottle in their hip pocket that the pharmacy ran out of penicillin! We are aware now that this method of use could sensitize a person to penicillin.

Compared to streptococcal infections, spirochetes are represented in only a small percent of the total number of dental infections. Even less involved, but nevertheless significant to patients when they occur, are infections from parasites.

Dr. Price reported a case in which a woman patient had a huge abscess in her neck from a fistula of a lower infected molar tooth. Even after the tooth was extracted, the chronic abscess resisted treatment efforts for many weeks. A bacterial examination disclosed the presence of a large number of amoeba. Treatment for amoebic parasites promptly stopped the infection.

On the following page are pictures of this woman's condition: the fistula draining under her chin, an x-ray picture showing her teeth and the infected tooth socket, plus a microscopic slide picture of the amoeba parasites causing her distress.

Amoeba were also found to nearly always be present in pyorrhea gum pockets and in at least one instance the parasite had penetrated into the adjacent bone. It is hoped that learning of the presence of such organisms and the local and systemic harm they can cause will stimulate all readers to seek regular, competent prophylaxis care by a dentist or dental hygienist every three to six months.

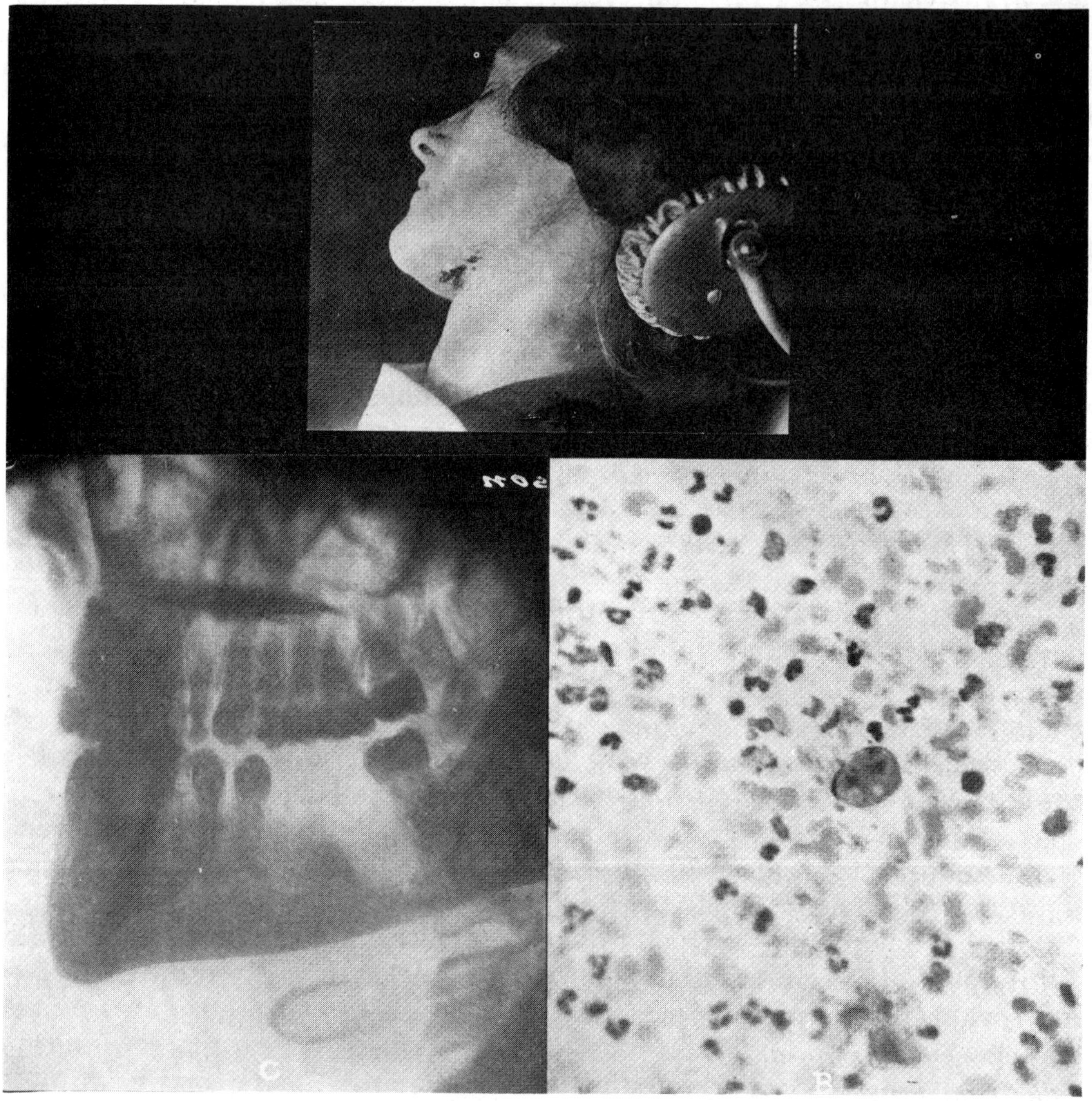

Pus draining fistula in A; infected tooth socket and large area of jaw bone loss; microscopic slide of large number of amoeba from infected area.

While the foremost difficulties investigated by Price concerned infections in the root canal and other tooth parts involving streptococcus organisms, in this chapter we have tried to point out some other organisms that can be responsible for systemic disease.

Bacteria can also be involved via the mouth in a few other ways. At the time of the Dr. Price studies, tuberculosis was a rather common serious illness. Dr. Price pointed out to his colleagues at the Research Institute that severe tooth decay areas that exposed the pulp could be providing an entry way through the teeth into the body for the tuberculosis bacillus. By traveling through the root canal into adjacent tissue, bacteria could be picked up by the lymphatic system and transported to the lymph glands of the neck, and from there to other body areas.

Enlarged cervical glands persisting for periods of time seemed to miraculously disappear when infected teeth were removed from patients, proving that bacteria do travel from the tooth to the neck.

Tuberculosis became a reasonably easy disease to treat when antibiotics arrived. Now, however, it is again attacking more and more people — and customary treatments aren't doing what they used to. The bacteria are mutating, changing their form and characteristics, much like what Price found to be occurring with organisms in dentin tubules.

Most people know that certain bacterial infections can be transmitted to others, such as scarlet fever, diphtheria, etc. Most also know that a person can be a carrier and transmit a disease without themselves being infected. *Do you suppose that those who have badly decayed teeth would be more apt to be carriers of bacterial infections? Don't you suppose that these people would also be more susceptible to becoming seriously infected themselves?*

Summary:

- The most prevalent organisms that inhabit the mouth were discussed and it was stated that of the 10 varieties of streptococcus bacteria, the "fecalis" family were predominant in 65 $^1/_2$ percent of the cases tested.

- This chapter deals with the spirochete species, amoeba parasite infections, and the tuberculosis bacillus.

- Although Dr. Price was able to demonstrate that a huge tumor-like mass on a rabbit's knee and a large thigh abscess resulted from the culture of spirochetes, he found systemic infections in laboratory animals from these bacteria occurred only rarely.

- Trench mouth, that is Vincent's infection, more commonly known today as acute necrotizing ulcerative gingivitis, is another matter. It is caused by a spirochete that is a cousin to the species that causes syphilis and appears together and acts jointly with a fusiform bacillus.

- Syphilis, in certain stages of the disease, does exhibit oral manifestations but its spirochetes are entirely different than the family of spirochetes involved in trench mouth.

- Trench mouth in its severe form can cause loss of teeth, debilitation, and loss of weight. It is related to poor dietary practices, deficiencies of vitamins B & C and certain minerals. The disease can be controlled with penicillin.

- My experiences with the use of penicillin in curing trench mouth during a World War II epidemic at an army air corps base were presented.

- Dentists generally have not been well acquainted with the role of spirochetes in the treatment of chronic periodontal gum disease. Dr. Price, in his bacteriologic studies, detected ten treponema spirochete species present in periodontal pockets. He admitted that the studies were not able to disclose which one or ones were primarily involved.

- Spirochete infections are involved in only a small percentage of dental infections and infections involving parasites are even less prevalent. Nevertheless they do occur.

- Pictures in this chapter of a huge abscess in the neck of a woman patient shows the socket and extensive area of jaw bone loss, and the pus draining fistula, plus the large number of amoeba present that caused the infection.

- Dr. Price's bacteriologic studies of the numbers of organisms in pyorrhea pockets almost always disclosed amoeba as well as bacteria.

- It was pointed out that a key benefit to having prophylaxis tooth cleaning every three to six months, in addition to preventing the need for root canal treatment, was the minimizing of bacteremias arising from the gum crevice areas.

- At the time of the Price studies, tuberculosis was a common serious illness. Dr. Price pointed out to his colleagues at the American Dental Association Research Institute that teeth with large open cavities exposing nerves and blood vessels of teeth could provide an easy entry way for the tuberculosis bacillus to be picked up by the lymphatic system, to be transported to the lymph glands of the neck, and to travel from there to other areas. "T.B." germs were easy to irradicate with antibiotics but they now mutate like those in root canals.

- Most dentists are quite familiar with enlarged cervical glands in the neck from dental infections and how they quickly disappear when infected teeth are removed.

- These various infections are additional reasons for people not to neglect their oral health.

CHAPTER 8

Mouth Bacteria Act and Perform Differently Than Other Organisms Their Jekyll and Hyde Lifestyle

We are all aware that the organisms that cause the breakout of mumps, typhoid fever, measles, diphtheria, smallpox, scarlet fever, etc. are highly specialized strains of certain infectious bacteria. On the other hand, organisms that are involved in dental infections, for the most part, do not target their activities against a specific organ or set of tissues. When they do, it is generally because the person infected has had, or is at the time suffering from, an acute process or difficulty in that tissue. Not only that, but when the cause of the focus of infection is removed — that is, the infected tooth, tonsil, tonsil tag, etc. — the acute process or illness usually completely disappears.

Strangely enough, streptococcus — and sometimes other organisms — as they originally appear in the mouth are relatively harmless, non-virulent strains of bacteria. What is so unique about these germs is their great capability of adapting to whatever confronts them in their environmental surroundings. Dr. Price found that they could learn to thrive and cause serious illnesses even in the presence of poisons which originally, in but one-tenth the concentration, would have completely inhibited their growth. *These same families of organisms did not have any of these destructive qualities when they first took up residence in the mouth.*

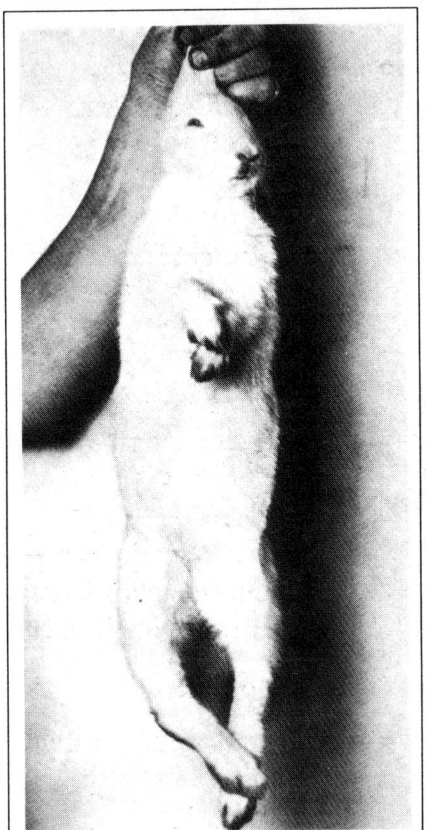

Extreme deforming arthritis from an implanted tooth of arthritic patient.

Earlier I stated that when the bacteria trapped in root filled teeth escape their nesting place in the tooth, they have a free ride in the bloodstream to any and all tissues of the body. *In their travels through the liver, heart, joints, eyes, kidneys, etc., certain bacteria will find one or more organs or tissues attractive and set up a new home life, a life that results in that tissue becoming disabled.*

In most cases, the patient's specific problem, such as rheumatism or arthritis, would flare up as the same disease in the rabbit after it had received an inoculation from the patient's infected tooth. Although this frequently proved to be the case, at times other tissues would become involved. Reviewing some of the case histories that Price reported makes it easier to understand how and why a rabbit developed a particular illness.

For example, a culture was made from an extracted root filled tooth taken from a patient with arthritis and subsequently four rabbits were inoculated with the bacteria. All four of the rabbits developed acute rheumatism but, in addition, two of them contracted liver trouble, one gallbladder lesions, one intestinal difficulty, and two developed brain lesions.

A second patient with acute rheumatism upset the health of nine rabbits in somewhat different ways: seven developed rheumatism, one liver trouble, two heart involvement, and one recovered.

In a third case, a patient who had myositis (muscle disturbance), neuritis, and lumbago was studied on two separate occasions. Of the three rabbits inoculated from the first extracted tooth, all three rabbits developed rheumatism, two heart lesions, one disease of the lungs, three of the liver, one gallbladder, two intestinal, and two kidney involvements. Added up, all these diseases seem to involve 14 rabbits, but actually all of them occurred in only the three that were inoculated. Patients likewise sometimes have two or more degenerative disease conditions.

The development of diseases in several other organs happened quite frequently to rabbits. Later, the same patient, who was not ill at the time, had another root filled tooth removed. It was cultured and bacteria inoculated into new rabbits. This time none developed rheumatism, but three did develop an acute liver condition and one a heart lesion.

In the beginning, Dr. Price introduced bacteria living in root filled teeth by implanting a tooth under a rabbit's skin. As time went on, he introduced organisms by imbedding just small pieces of a tooth's root, or by powdering the roots and injecting the powder. Eventually, bacteria were transferred from the teeth and grown in a culture medium, and thereafter the bacteria were injected into rabbits for investigative purposes. Each method caused similar degenerative diseases.

Another acute rheumatism case caused 10 inoculated rabbits to experience disease conditions in the following tissues: three in the heart, three in lungs, three liver, two stomach, four in the kidneys, five developed rheumatism, and one myositis. After the tooth extraction, this patient had no recurrence of her previous troubles in the three years that she was studied.

Inoculations from patients having acute eye problems caused a high percentage of eye trouble to develop in rabbits. One patient had exophthalmos (protruding eyes) and was also suffering from extreme pain from the rupturing of blood vessels. The inoculation of 13 rabbits with that patient's culture resulted in 62 percent developing eye involvements, 69 percent intestinal and digestion tract lesions, and the occurrence of a number of other severe tissue lesions.

The culture from a patient totally blind in one eye and having four-fifths loss of sight in the other caused one rabbit to develop multiple lesions and the other nine to experience eye trouble.

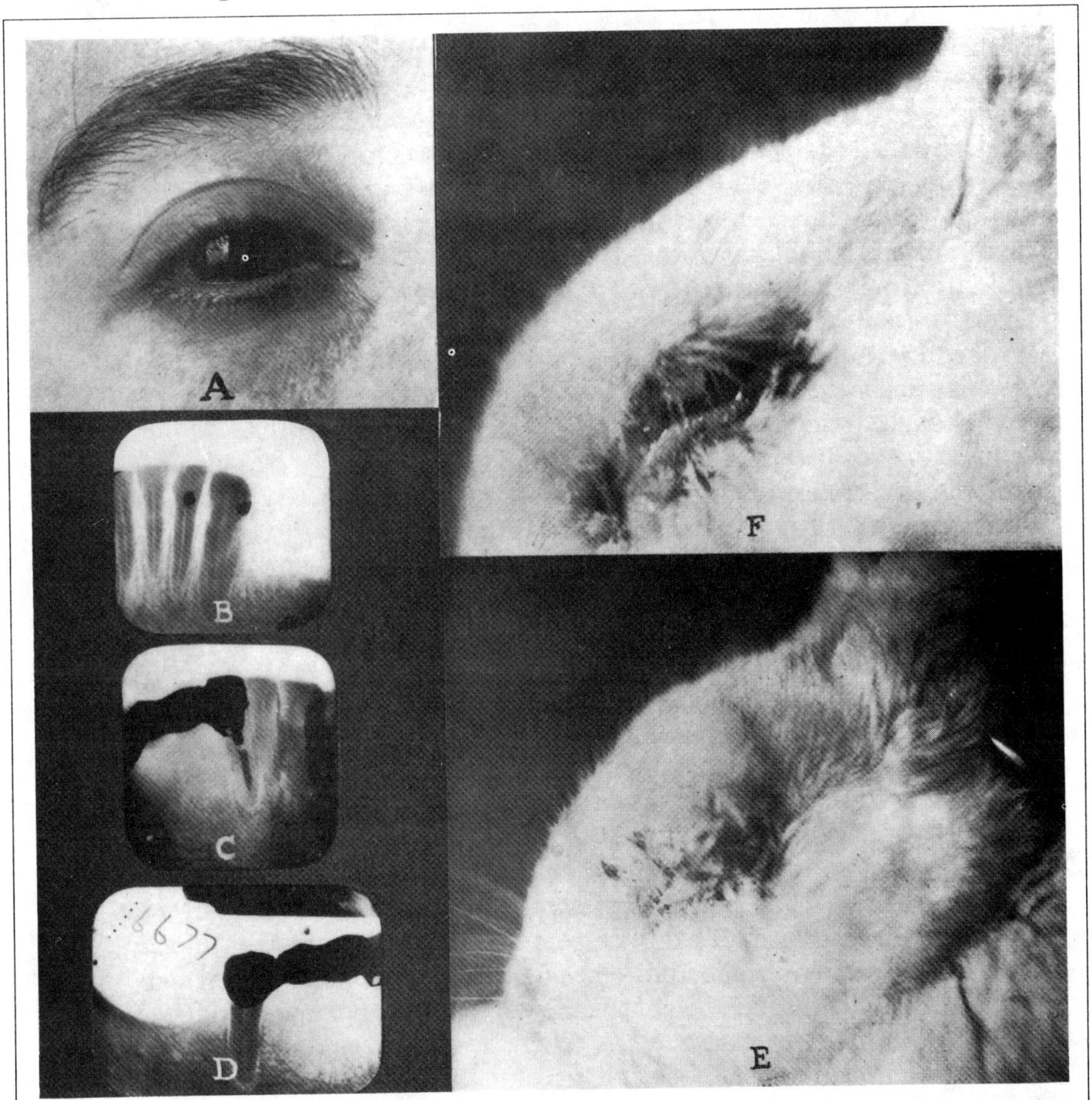

Extreme eye involvement of Case No. 861. B, C and D: dental conditions. E and F: progressive stages of acute involvement in the eye of a rabbit that had been inoculated with a culture from the teeth shown in B, C and D.

Regarding a patient suffering from diarrhea and bowel movements every 15 minutes, all of four rabbits developed diarrhea. In another acute digestive case, of six inoculated rabbits, three had involvement of their stomachs and intestines, and one of the gallbladder and liver. After that effort, the cultured material was passed through a Berkefeld filter to remove all bacteria, leaving only their toxins. These toxins were then inoculated into nine rabbits: 44 percent developed intestinal trouble, 67 percent liver disturbances, and 33 percent heart diseases, proving that the by-products of bacteria are as dangerous, if not more so, than the organisms themselves.

You can see from all these cases that more often than not rabbits developed the patient's disease when inoculated. At the same time, it wasn't unusual for them to become victims of diseases in a number of other organs or tissues. In a few instances, the rabbits didn't exhibit the patient's illness but developed an entirely different disease.

It should be stated again that Dr. Price found that acute processes usually did not develop in rabbits when organisms were taken from teeth at a time when the patient was not suffering from any infirmity.

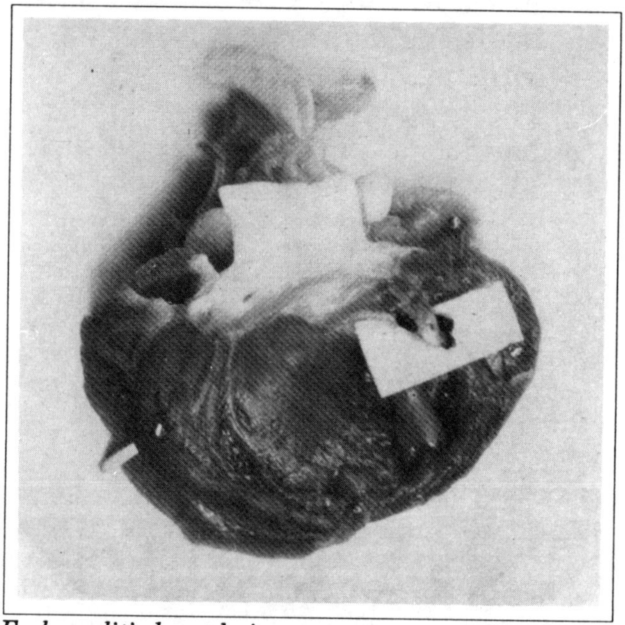

Endocarditis heart lesion.

Patients who had root canal fillings but didn't become ill were found to have particularly good defense mechanisms that controlled bacteria and thereby prevented infections from being transferred to their organs and tissues. In other words, their white blood cells and other immune system activities were able to engulf and control the number of bacteria that were escaping from their teeth.

Summary:

- The organisms that cause dental infections do not generally direct their activities toward any specific organ or tissue as do the bacteria strains that are responsible for the outbreak of measles, mumps, smallpox, diphtheria, etc.

- When dental infections seem to target a specific organ or set of tissues, that patient often proves to have had a prior history of difficulty in that tissue or is currently having trouble.

- When the cause of an illness is focal infection from a tooth, tonsil, tonsil tag, or other area and that source of infection is removed, the acute process usually disappears. When the cause of the illness is not from a focal infection source, it does not go away upon such removal.

- The organisms that live in the mouth on a day-to-day basis are harmless and non-poisonous. However, when the teeth or mouth tissues become diseased, these same bacteria have the ability to adapt, mutate, and thrive, often causing serious illnesses even in the presence of disinfectants that at one-tenth the concentration would have previously killed them.

- Most often rabbits would develop the same disease as the patient but in many instances they developed additional diseases. Some examples of actual cases follow:
  * Patient with arthritis — Bacteria isolated from the extracted teeth were inoculated into four rabbits. All four developed severe rheumatism. In addition, two developed liver trouble, one gallbladder lesions, one intestinal difficulties, and two developed brain lesions.
  * Patient with acute rheumatism — Nine rabbits were inoculated with bacteria from the root filled tooth. Seven developed rheumatism, one liver trouble, two heart involvements, and one recovered.
  * Patient with myositis (muscle disturbance), neuritis, and lumbago — Three rabbits were inoculated with bacteria from the extracted tooth. All three developed rheumatism, two heart lesions, one disease of the lungs, three of the liver, one gallbladder, two intestinal, and two kidney involvement. A total of 14 conditions took place in the three rabbits.
  * I won't summarize the many other examples discussed in this chapter other than to say that they involved, in addition to the above named organs, the stomach, kidneys, eyes, and gastro intestinal tract.

- It was felt that Dr. Price implanted whole teeth under the skin of rabbits because he wasn't sure where the infection was located in the teeth.

- While some people viewed the above as a crude procedure, it produced the same result as making a culture of a diseased area in order to develop a vaccine; testing the ability of drugs to kill bacteria; or transmitting the disease to animals in order to test treatment methods.

- After imbedding whole teeth, Dr. Price used small pieces of the tooth's root instead, and later the roots were powdered and the powder injected. Eventually bacteria from the teeth were cultured and then the bacteria that were isolated were injected into the rabbit.

- Each of these methods proved to be ways that would disclose the presence of infections in root canal filled teeth — teeth that appeared to be sound and healthy.

- *It is interesting to note that if patients with root canal fillings were not experiencing any health problems and had these teeth extracted, the rabbits that were inoculated with the products of such teeth usually did not develop any infirmities.*

- It was surmised that the good defense mechanisms of these patients were able to control the bacteria and the toxins present in the dentin tubules. This occurred because their bodies were not overburdened by other debilitating conditions and, in addition, they had white blood cells and other body defender mechanisms ready and able to engulf the bacteria and their toxins as they move into the bloodstream from the dentin tubules.

- The rabbits inoculated from these teeth didn't develop illness because the numbers of bacteria and toxins were much diminished by the patient's immune system.

CHAPTER 9

Root Canal Fillings Getting Better but Still a Problem

After pulp and infected material has been removed from the inside of an infected tooth and the area sterilized, the root canal is filled. The intention when placing a root filling is to fill the canal completely to the very end of the root. Dentists attempt to do this accurately since it is well-known that an incompletely filled canal, or one that lacks solidarity, is prone to allow bacteria present in the bloodstream to enter those unfilled areas and become a source of reinfection.

Most root canal treated teeth today are expertly filled. Below you see two that are excellent and two that are inadequate.

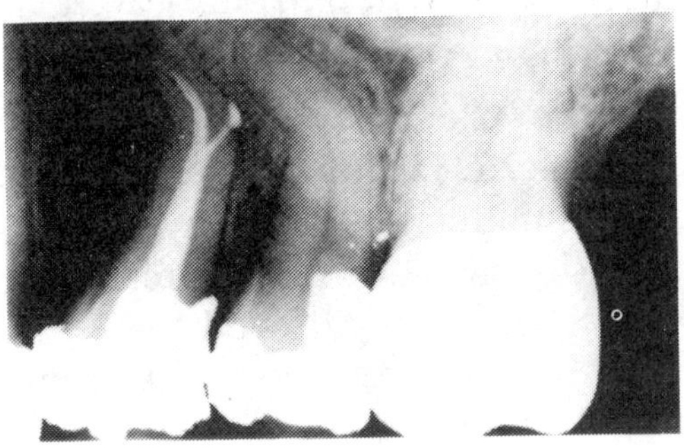

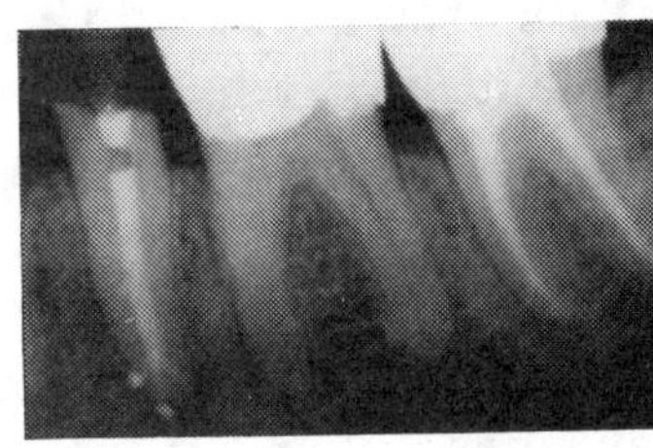

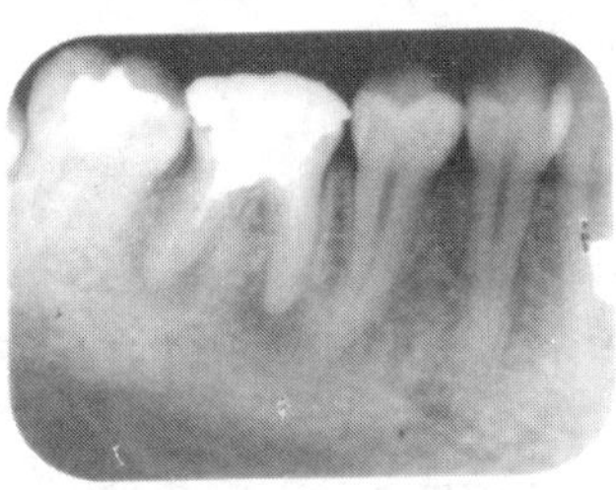

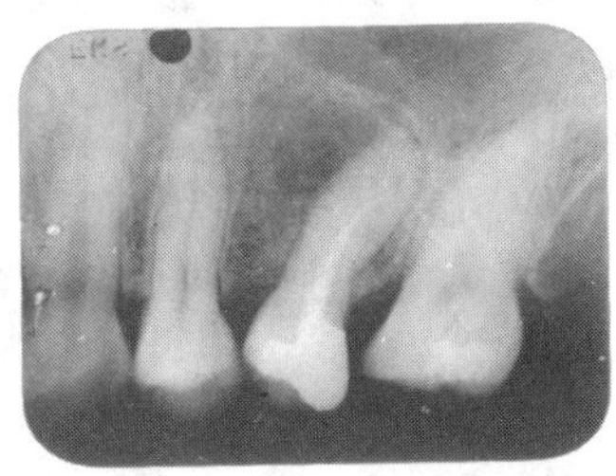

In his research investigations of root filling materials, Dr. Price was able to call upon his previous experience gained during prior studies of dental waxes, gold, and other materials used in dental work. These studies are equally as important as the study of root filling materials for these materials also must be able to be applied accurately if dentists are to make correct fitting castings of inlays and crowns. Dr. Price found and reported in scientific dental journals that dental waxes had great variations in dimensions and casting gold shrunk two percent in mass in going from a liquid to solid state, as did root canal filling materials.

It was this background that led Dr. Price to an investigation of the expansion and contraction of gutta-percha, the most widely used root filling material. Gutta-percha is a rubbery-like substance that packs more easily if it is somewhat warmed. However, when it cools and sets for a few days, shrinkage does take place.

To test dimensional change, Dr. Price devised a way to pack gutta-percha into small glass tubes using a metal piston he invented which exerted a force of over several hundred pounds pressure to pack and condense the material. The gutta-percha was tested at several different degrees of temperature and the piston of the packer was set to keep a steady, heavy pressure on the gutta-percha in order to minimize the shrinkage problem, something that could not be done in the mouth.

When the root filling material had cooled sufficiently, the exposed end of the tube was submerged into a liquid blue dye. In every test, the gutta-percha leaked, that is shrank away from the glass walls and the ink traveled up through this area and into the material. His pictures of these tests clearly demonstrate that it was impossible to pack gutta-percha at a temperature that permitted it to be molded without the ink flowing into it, meaning that bacteria could live in these spaces.

Another widely used method was also investigated. Both chloroform and eucalyptol are solvents of gutta-percha. If gutta-percha is allowed to completely dissolve in either of these liquids and the cream mass that results is allowed to set, the mass shrinks two-thirds as the liquid evaporates.

The mixture of gutta-percha and chloroform is called chlorapercha. Because this mixture has a certain ideal stickiness to it, another technique for filling a tooth canal was to moisten standard gutta-percha that filled a canal to 90 percent of its size with the chlorapercha, trusting that it would fill the remaining 10 percent of the space. Price found that in such cases, when the moisture of the chloroform evaporated, the canal still lacked 6.6 percent of being full. Not only that, the stickiness subsided and the material pulled away from the tooth.

Dentists have used this method, along with pressure packing, to try to overcome the shrinkage problem. Today, numbers of other root filling pastes have been made available and most contain some type of disinfectant in an attempt to ensure the killing of bacteria. Gutta-percha is still widely used and tests by other investigators confirm the difficulty that exists of completely filling the canal, no matter what filling material is used.

The intent of a fairly recent study reported in the *Journal of Endodontia* in 1984 was to examine and overcome shrinkage problems inherent to root canal filling materials and was carried out by dentists Torabinejad, Kahn, and Bankes using isopropyl cyanoacrylate as a root canal sealer. Along with this new material, they investigated three popular commercial sealers.

The cyanoacrylate sealer was introduced into the root canal with a syringe rather than applied by the usual file method. A gutta-percha fitted point was used as the root canal filling material using lateral condensation. Leakage was determined by immersing the root tips in India ink for 24 hours.

Dr. Louis Grossman, Endodontic Professor, in discussing root canal sealers stated that the following characteristics are essential: tackiness for adherence to root canal walls; ability to completely seal the canal; radiopaqueness; ability to mix easily with cement; lack of shrinkage when set; does not stain teeth; bacteriostatic; slow setting; insoluble in tissue fluids; biocompatible; and soluble in common solvents should removal of filling materials become necessary.

Torabinejad, Kahn and Banks rightly felt that isopropyl cyanoacrylate has good potential as a sealer as its 0.5mm leakage proved so superior to other materials tested. These investigators should be commended for recognizing the importance of obliterating the root canal and in working toward a technique to make it impermeable to bacteria. Though the measured leakage they achieved was cut down to 0.5mm of space, that still represents a significant area for organisms to accumulate.

These leaking areas in and around root canal fillings provide a cave-like dwelling area in which bacteria can reside. Such areas are, in effect, a walled-in fortress in which organisms can survive until they find a means to sneak back into general circulation or back into the canal. At the same time, because the normal blood supply to the inside of the tooth no longer exists, there is no way for the cells of the immune system to get in and attack bacteria hiding out in these spaces.

In spite of all of these difficulties, many people have been free from these secondary infections of teeth because they happen to be blessed with immune systems that are able to satisfactorily control the organisms and thereby prevent a degenerative disease takeover.

One other somewhat related investigation was undertaken by Dr. Price; that was to determine if teeth that contained root fillings and were sterile would keep their sterility. In this study *healthy* extracted teeth were root filled outside of the mouth using sterile techniques. They were found to have remained sterile for two or more weeks. At that point the outside of these teeth were contaminated by subjecting them to a culture medium that contained pathogenic bacteria. The test was made to see if bacteria would penetrate the outside surfaces of the tooth and travel inwardly to the root canal. In most instances, in but a few weeks time, the organisms were found inside the tooth structure and in or beside the root filling material, thereby proving that bacteria could find their way through the lateral accessory canals and the dentin tubules back into the tooth.

To conclude this chapter, I directly quote Dr. Price regarding the efficiency of root canal fillings:

> *"When we consider how many thousands of the extracted teeth we have cultured and found to be infected within the tooth structure, and the extremely low percentage, practically zero, in which infection was not demonstrated, together with the fact that so many teeth with excellent root fillings show structural changes of the supporting tissues after a few years have elapsed, we are led to believe that* ***root fillings rarely fill pulp canals sufficiently perfectly to shut out bacteria completely. Root fillings usually fill the pulp canal much less perfectly some time after the operation, than at the time of the operation, due to the contraction of the root filling material. The ultimate volume contraction of the root filling is approximately the amount of solvent used where a solvent is used with gutta-percha as a root filling material."***

In spite of all this, Dr. Price, as he did many times in some form, stated:

> *"It is not proven that it is absolutely necessary that teeth be perfectly sterilized or that they be perfectly root filled in order that an individual may not develop systemic involvement, since under favorable conditions the patient may provide an adequate defense or quarantine against these organisms."*

Summary:

- The perfect filling of a root canal should completely fill and seal the canal to the very tip of the root.

- With all the research that has gone on by untold numbers of investigators, this ideal has yet to be accomplished.

- Keep in mind that any space not occupied by the root canal filling can be contaminated by the ingress of bacteria that are often present in the bloodstream and by bacteria present in dentin tubules.

- The fact that 30 percent of people with root canal fillings were free of complicating degenerative diseases does not alter the concern about the continuing presence of bacteria in their root filled teeth. To the 70 percent who are suffering health problems, inadequately filled root canals add insult to injury.

- Most of the spaces remaining after filling are due to shrinkage of the root filling material.

- Gutta percha, still the most widely used root filling material, was scientifically tested by Dr. Price using a packing device he invented to eliminate usual packing technique difficulties, yet not a single test filling was free of leakage.

- A 1984 report in the *Journal of Endodontia* of a new material, cyanoacrylate used along with gutta-percha, found leakage cut down to 0.5 millimeters of space. Though a big improvement, that still represents a significant cave-like dwelling area for organisms to accumulate, from which bacteria can sneak back into the general circulation and cause body harm.

- Dr. Price did devise a test using healthy extracted teeth that demonstrated how these spaces in root fillings, even if sterile initially, could become infected from blood circulation.

- Dr. Price did state that neither root fillings nor sterilization procedures needed to be perfect providing the patient's immune system was adequate enough to meet such challenges.

CHAPTER 10

Gum Infections, Like Those of Teeth, Can Cause Destructive Body Ailments

Over the years, infections of the gums have been known by several names, commonly: periodontal disease, periodontoclasia, and pyorrhea alveolaris.

Dr. Price stated that he could not find, in all of medicine — including dental medicine, any common diseases that so baffled explanation or which contained so many paradoxes as has the disease of the gums.

Even though much research effort has been expended since Dr. Price's time on the various factors of disease of the gums, and because one-third of my own dental practice days were spent treating periodontal illness, it is with some difficulty that I tell you that there still exists a wide divergence of opinion and confusion as to just what this condition is all about.

Most dentists seem to be in agreement now that the irritation of the rough tartar deposits (calculus) that accumulate in the gum crevices causes the gum tissue to become inflamed and to attract bacteria. When these deposits are not thoroughly scaled off the teeth by a dental hygienist or dentist, more and more calculus accumulates and more and more bacteria gather and live in the gum crevice. As the process continues, there occurs a gradual destruction of the gum fibers that hold the gum to the tooth. This is accompanied by an eating away of the bone that supports the tooth, an accumulation of even greater numbers of bacteria, and a foulness of the breath.

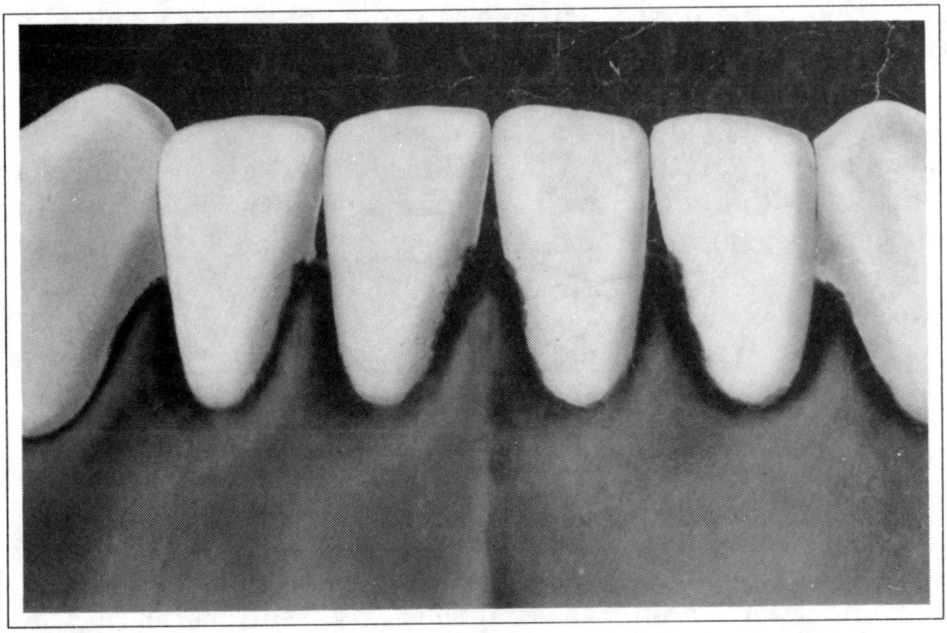

Periodontal disease. Tarter deposits forming in gum crevices. Gums irritated, swollen, inflamed.

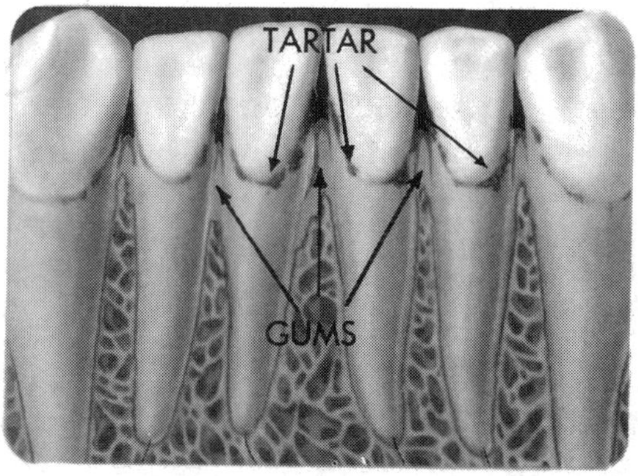

When tartar is not removed regularly, gums recede, deep pockets form, bacteria accumulate.

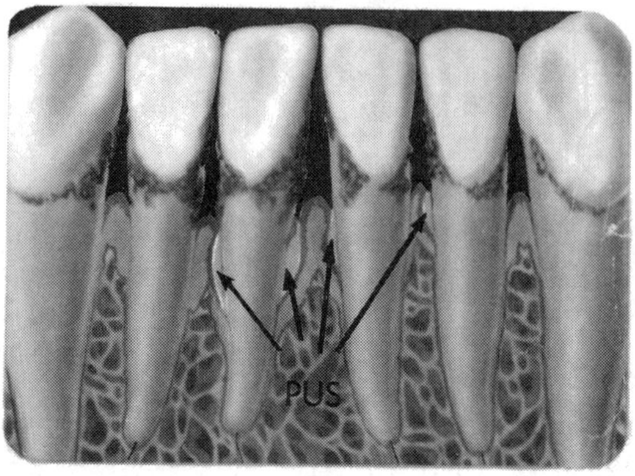

Pyorrhea pockets. Much deeper bacteria growth, heavy pus flows, teeth begin to loosen.

If treatment is not instituted, the teeth will lose their bony support and eventually become very loose, and if not extracted, will fall out of their own accord.

Dr. Price held views regarding pyorrhea similar to those above, saying that these were the beliefs of his time — but he added that the success of the removal of the various irritants did not explain the cause of the disease. He even stated that traumatic bite problems are irritants and that they too must be corrected. The fact that he recognized bite problems as a contributing factor so long ago is extraordinary as this had been given little attention until more recent times.

In trying to understand the various causative problems involved in periodontal disease, he studied the different theories and found only confusion and contradiction. Dr. Price then instigated an intensive investigation and study of this dental disease.

He took a new approach, one that included an exhaustive analysis of clinical data and a thorough, careful examination of the characteristics present in those people with the disease. He then related the information collected to the patients' blood and saliva chemistrys and to the bacteria that he found present.

For a long time Dr. Price could not accept the findings of his own studies as they seemed so paradoxical and far-fetched. In the close study of some 1400 cases, he eventually classified dental infections into three main categories and a few subdivisions.

These studies indicated that a person's biological inheritance played a major role as the disease was more likely to occur in those who had one or both parents with pyorrhea.

Another important finding was that the early treatment of periodontal disease resulted in a complete cure, providing that all tartar deposits and/or ill fitting fillings were replaced. In advanced cases of pyorrhea, if the removal of the irritants was the only treatment employed, much less improvement took place.

With local topical treatment of early cases with medications, even when irritating deposits were not removed, there was also marked improvement. Cases treated by the injection of bactericidal drugs likewise resulted in improvement when early treatment of the disease was undertaken.

On the other hand, when more supporting bone was lost and the pyorrhea pockets became deeper, the overall conditions and outlook changed remarkably. The surprise was the number of systemic body changes that were found to take place. Among them were the considerable amount of absorption of bone; the occurrence or non-occurrence of dental caries (cavities); changes in the uric acid level; and, in addition, changes in the blood and saliva of the ionic calcium level, and its urea nitrogen content.

In time it became apparent that the presence or absence of gum infections was directly related to the patient's calcium metabolism. When the ionic level of calcium in the blood was higher than normal, the supporting gum and bone tended to be absorbed away more easily in the presence of irritation.

At the same time, studies of saliva revealed it to be more alkaline than usual when periodontal disease was active. Another big surprise occurred when the contents of the pus pockets were found to be very alkaline, having a pH as high as 7.7, when dentists would assume it to be acid. The pH of the blood and saliva when normal is 7.4.

One would think that when teeth affected by periodontal disease are extracted there would be some difficulties with healing. Quite the contrary, sockets developed good blood clots and healed rapidly, without pain or the development of a dry socket.

On the other hand, those cases that were marked by the formation of the dense bone of condensing osteitis below the tooth's root end proved to be painful, healed slowly, developed blood clots that easily broke down, and many of these cases exhibited the dreaded dry socket. An analysis of the saliva of such patients showed it to be lower in alkalinity and the blood lower in ionic calcium.

It should be more apparent now that the cases mentioned involve two distinct types of individuals. This was borne out even more dramatically when two different types of extraction sockets were examined under a microscope. Here too, the disparity proved so definite as to be of diagnostic value.

The sockets of teeth extracted because of pyorrhea were found to contain primarily polymorphonuclear white blood cells having several lobes. Many granules (granulocytes) were seen under the microscope and these cells showed rapid movements. The white cells were seen to be doing their work of engulfing the bacteria and only a few of the organisms escaped entrapment.

Sockets of teeth extracted for root end infections when condensing osteitis was present had only a few white blood cells (leucocytes) and granules, but large numbers of organisms outside these cells.

These research efforts demonstrated that as alkalinity went down, ionic calcium levels went up. Such cases were accompanied by acute inflammatory reactions to irritation agents with destruction of gum attachments and absorption of alveolar bone.

Dentists looked upon pyorrhea as being primarily an infectious disease at the time of the Price studies, and many still do today. You can see from the data that, although bacteria are present, pyorrhea is not due to a specific infection but, rather, involves definite systemic body conditions. The factors were found to be related to a person's specific susceptibility and biological inheritance; that is, they are connected in a very definite way to one's own biological defense and ability of the immune system.

Those of us involved in the nutritional background of dental disease have argued for many years about the relation of calcium, phosphorus, other minerals, and certain vitamins to the causes of gum disease and tooth decay. Many leading periodontists have scoffed at these assertions, stating that all that is needed to cure such conditions is good dental treatment or dental surgery.

You can readily see from the results of Dr. Price's thorough research that any number of body systems are involved in such diseases. The large number of individuals who end up losing all of their teeth could be reduced in the future by consideration of the systemic problems that are involved.

Summary:

- Diseases of the gums baffle explanation and contain many paradoxes.

- Though much research has gone on since Price's time, many opposing views still exist, resulting in confusion about gum diseases.

- Periodontal disease, commonly called pyorrhea, is the result of the accumulation of tartar deposits in the gum crevice. When not removed regularly and thoroughly every three to six months by a hygienist or dentist, the rough character of the deposits and the bacteria they harbor cause destruction of the gum's attachment to the tooth and to the bone that holds teeth in place.

- Removal of deposits and various other irritants does not really explain the cause of the disease. Price pondered the confusion and contradictions and decided on taking a new approach.

- This involved an exhaustive investigation and study of the clinical data available; a careful examination of the characteristics of those having this dental disease; blood and saliva chemistry information; and the relationship of these findings to the bacteria present. Close study of some 1400 cases was undertaken.

- These studies indicated that inheritance had much to do with whether or not a person developed pyorrhea, as Dr. Price found pyorrhea more prevalent in those with one or both parents having the disease.

- It is my view that this factor may be largely an environmental one as dietary habits of a patient's parents are often similar to that of the patient, especially in formative years. Tooth decay, for example, is more prevalent in a child who follows the diet of a parent who eats an excess of sweets.

- Dr. Price's in-depth studies of saliva and blood indicated that the occurrence of periodontal gum infections was directly related to calcium metabolism. Later research by Harold Hawkins, D.D.S. in Los Angeles during the 1930s and 1940s found infections to be related to the calcium-phosphorous balance, as have others. Disclosures resulting from these studies, in addition to those related to changes in ionic calcium values that occurred in both blood and saliva, were:
  * Changes in the uric acid level;
  * Change in the urea nitrogen content;
  * Saliva became more alkaline when periodontal disease was active;
  * Contents of pus pockets became very alkaline, although dentists would suppose them to be more acid;
  * When teeth affected by periodontal disease were extracted, healing was rapid and without pain or the development of a dry socket;
  * However, if condensing osteitis — that is, dense bone below the root end was present, healing became slow, painful, and a dry socket was more likely to develop. Saliva became lower in alkalinity and the ionic calcium level in blood also proved to be lower.

- Because treatment of periodontal disease by competent dentists generally achieves such good results, periodontists often deny findings such as those made by Dr. Price. While getting rid of the infected tissue can lead to the impression of a cure, readers and dentists alike must come to terms with the knowledge that there are many systemic factors that ought to be changed if return of the disease is to be prevented.

CHAPTER 11

Life in Every Form Seems Dependent Upon Ionic Calcium

Of all the numerous investigations that were made by Dr. Price, the one that produced the most confusion and required the most research time was his investigation into the role of calcium. He states that every cell of the body is dependent on the presence of ionic calcium. It is used in teeth and bones, in the movement of muscles, in the rhythmic action of the heart and intestines, and is indispensable for the coagulation of blood at the time of cuts, injuries, surgeries, etc.

And that is only part of the story. In addition to these important functions, Dr. Price found calcium to have a remarkable role to play when infections are present, in metabolism, during pregnancy, in the maintenance of the acid-alkaline balance of the body, in the presence or absence of tooth decay, pyorrhea and other degenerative diseases, and that it should be given more consideration in studies of immunity and susceptibility.

It was a great disappointment to Dr. Price that medical literature contained so little information about these critical problems and it was partially due to this deficiency that Dr. Price embarked on his own many pursuits of the subject. To make matters worse, dental pathology in literature was filled with paradoxes, many directly or indirectly related to calcium in both negative and positive ways.

A couple of puzzling key situations were (1) the wasting away of bone surrounding teeth in cases of pyorrhea and (2) the large areas of bone eaten away at the root ends of infected teeth. Individuals having these conditions were found to have high amounts of ionic calcium. In such instances, one is more apt to expect the calcium level to be low rather than high.

A similar situation existed in rheumatoid arthritis cases that were marked by loss of bone in the finger joints and other skeletal areas, and conversely with the building up of bone that occurs in osteoarthritis cases. Where bone is lost, one would expect low ionic calcium to be the case but, instead, these patients proved to have high amounts of ionic calcium. Conversely, one would expect thick bony areas and the building of bone in osteoarthritics to be high in ionic calcium, but these patients were found to have low amounts of ionic calcium in the blood.

Whenever your physician or dentist has a blood panel test run, two of the items that will be determined are the amount of calcium and the amount of phosphorus in your blood. Most medical laboratories state the normal value of calcium to be 8.5 to 10.5 mg/dl and the phosphorus 2.5 to 4.5 mg/dl.

Many laboratories now also list the amount of ionic calcium; that is, the amount of calcium carrying an electric charge. While many doctors roughly estimate the ionic calcium to be about half of the total amount of calcium that is shown in the blood test, this can be quite inaccurate.

Of that normal 10 to 10.7 mg of calcium, approximately four milligrams are actually a part of the protein enzyme thrombin that plays an active role in the clotting of blood. Less than a milligram of the normal 10 mg/dl is contained in our various blood cells. The remaining five milligrams of the total are ionic calcium.

The calcium in thrombin is relatively constant in order to assure the clotting of blood and must be there to prevent our bleeding to death. If your blood panel amount of calcium turns out to be low, say 7.5 mg/dl, when you subtract the 4 mg of calcium present in the thrombin and the 1 mg contained in blood cells, the amount remaining as ionized calcium would only be 2.5 mg. It is by understanding this body mechanism and function that you will appreciate what Dr. Price is referring to when he mentions low or high levels of ionic calcium.

Incidentally, physicians don't see the significance of these changes unless the calcium gets above 11 or 12 mg/dl, or lower than 8.5. When calcium is that high, they look for hyperparathyroidism, bony metastasis, too much vitamin D, cancer, long-term diuretic use, acidosis, or dehydration. When calcium is very low, doctors are concerned about hypoparathyroidism, malabsorption, pancreatitis, kidney failure, osteomalacia, rickets, and alkalosis.

The late Melvin Page, D.D.S. of St. Petersburg Beach, Florida was a great follower of Price's work in reference to the focal infections caused by teeth, tonsils, and tonsil tags, and also to Price's investigations into calcium. Dr. Page added much to Dr. Price's studies with his own blood studies, and research on the calcium/phosphorus balance and its relationship to virtually all disease conditions.

He showed that in order for us to utilize 10 mg of calcium, there has to be 4 mg of phosphorus present in the blood. Any amount less or more than 4 mg would contribute to body degeneration. This doesn't mean that calcium has to be exactly 10 mg and phosphorus 4; what is essential is that calcium be 2.5 times that of phosphorus.

In thousands and thousands of tests, Page found that the diets of most Americans cause them to have significant imbalances between calcium and phosphorus. The key dietary factors that put these two important elements out of balance are sugar, caffeine products, refined grains, and soft drinks.

For example, one teaspoonful of sugar or a cup of coffee causes the calcium in the body to go up and the phosphorus to go down. If you use sugar every day and a test is run of your blood, it will show that the amount of calcium will be elevated, perhaps to 10.8, and the phosphorus will have become lowered to a possible 3.4 mg. Now multiply the phosphorus you have by 2.5

and you will see that the amount of calcium that can actually be utilized is 8.5. But your blood test indicates that you have 10.8 mg of calcium present. By subtracting the 8.5 you can utilize from the 10.8 you have (10.8 - 8.5 = 2.30), you are left with 2.30 mg. That means there is 2.30 mg of calcium floating around in your bloodstream that your body cannot put into use. Such calcium that is traveling in every 100 mg of your blood that can't be utilized actually becomes toxic to the body tissues.

At this point, the questions you should be mulling over are: (1) Where does extra calcium come from? and (2) What can this extra calcium do to one's body? Nature provided you with a huge storage warehouse for just such emergencies: your skeleton. That extra calcium is pulled from your bones.

Keep in mind, calcium that can't be used because of insufficient phosphorus acts as a foreign toxic substance that can end up being deposited in body tissues. Such free calcium becomes a pathologic substance. For example, it can become deposits that show up in arthritic joints, or stones in the kidneys or gall bladder, the calcium in the elbow or shoulder when bursitis and tendonitis are present, the cataract in the eye, and it becomes the main constituent that builds up in arteries. You are never told, but the build-up in arteries in atherosclerosis is composed of 95 percent calcium and only 0.5 percent cholesterol.

With soft drinks, the opposite chemistry takes place inasmuch as these drinks are primarily composed of phosphoric acid plus some sweeteners and chemicals. The figures after drinking a soft drink look like this: calcium, instead of 10 goes down to 9.6, and phosphorus rises to 4.9. Multiply the amount of phosphorus 4.9 x 2.5 = 12.25 mg. This is the amount of calcium the phosphorus needs to keep it in balance. But you only have 9.60 mg of calcium, so that means you have 2.65 mg of free phosphorus floating around in your blood looking for calcium. It finds the calcium ready and waiting, available in your bones. Now if that only happens once in a while, there will be no problem as our bones are sufficiently dense and numerous enough to support occasional deficits of this kind. However, if these imbalances happen day after day, it can be a prime factor in the development of rheumatoid arthritis, rickets, osteoporosis, and osteomalacia.

Dr. Melvin Page found that whenever he was able to get patients to achieve a calcium balance that was two and one-half times that of their phosphorus, their degenerative diseases just disappeared. He authored three books but the data mentioned above was best covered in his popular best seller, *Young Minds With Old Bodies*.

Let's get back to Price's finding about how infections influenced the calcium balance. He, too, was concerned about the nutritional implications and sensed its importance in stating: *"The evidence on hand would seem to suggest that in most cases it is not so much the presence or absence of an available supply of calcium, such as calcium bearing foods, as it is* ***a disturbance of the mechanism which governs calcium metabolism****."*

He demonstrated the relationship that exists between thyroid and parathyroid activity in certain of his dental infection experiments. His many studies convinced him that the body's defense system could be enhanced by modifying calcium metabolism. At the same time, he made it known that the mechanisms for doing so were not yet clear. His later nutrition research into the diets of primitives did much to clarify how calcium and phosphorus function.

Dr. Weston Price's experiments kept going on day after day, year after year, for over twenty-five years! His serious, remarkable research proves to be far-reaching in every division of the subject of dentistry. Yet none of his discoveries were more startling or enlightening than those involving the significant changes produced in the blood and tissues of patients and animals from dental infections. Among his more important discoveries are the following:

Regarding Low Ionic Calcium

- Dental focal infections, in many instances, lower the ionic calcium level of the blood.
- When an infected tooth of a patient having a degenerative illness is placed in a vessel of the patient's blood, the ionic calcium drops markedly.
- Patients having degenerative diseases have low levels of ionic calcium and the total of the combined calcium present is also very low. However, when dental infections are removed, the balance is restored and ill health symptoms of patients usually progressively disappear.
- When an infected tooth of a patient was placed under the skin of a rabbit, the animal experienced a similar reduced ionic calcium of its blood and malfunctions of the glands of internal secretion were produced.
- When organisms originating from infected teeth were grown in culture and injected into animals, they produced changes in the animal's blood including a reduction in ionic calcium.
- Tooth decay occurs when the ionic calcium level is below normal.
- When ionic calcium levels are persistently low, such individuals have denser bones and they have difficulty responding to local anesthetics.
- Those with persistently low ionic calcium levels tend to have slow healing and repair and are likely to develop secondary infections of sockets following extractions.
- At those times when ionic calcium is low, patients are more apt to develop a dry socket after tooth extraction.
- People with low ionic calcium and condensing osteitis tend, after tooth extractions, to have spicules of bone work loose from the socket.

- Individuals having persistently low ionic calcium generally do not develop periodontal gum diseases.
- Individuals with high ionic calcium of the blood tend, quite regularly, to develop periodontal disease; whereas patients with low ionic calcium do not tend toward the development of gum diseases.
- When infected teeth are placed under the skin of rabbits, there is practically always a reduction of the ionic calcium of the rabbits' blood, and as death approaches, their ionic calcium levels decrease progressively. This generally occurs when the calcium gets to a low of 6 or 7 milligrams.

Regarding High Ionic Calcium Levels

- When patients have a liberal loss of bone from dental infections, they will generally have a high ionic calcium level in the blood.
- People who have freedom from tooth decay generally have ionic calcium level of the blood that is normal or above normal.
- Individuals who usually have high ionic calcium levels of the blood tend to have bones that are looser knit and less dense. They respond readily to local anesthetics.
- Low ionic calcium individuals tend to have slow healing and repair and have a marked tendency to secondary infections of sockets following extraction.
- People having high ionic calcium levels rarely have condensing osteitis or spicules of bone work loose after tooth extractions.
- Individuals with high ionic calcium levels of the blood quite regularly develop periodontal disease.

Other Blood Systemic Changes

- Dental infections reduce the body's normal alkalinity reserve in the blood of patients and animals.
- The removal of infected teeth in some individuals results in an improvement of the blood sugar relationship.
- The presence of dental infections increases the uric acid of the blood.

To conclude this chapter, it can be said that:

A. Life in every form appears to be dependent upon free ionic calcium.
B. The functions of cells — whether excessive, below normal activity, or in dysfunction — are either affected or directly controlled by the concentration of ionic calcium.
C. A person's vital capacity and vital efficiency are both inseparable from and dependent upon calcium metabolism.

D. Most of these various discoveries will be as new to dentists today as they were when Weston Price reported them.

Summary:

- The subject that occupied most of Dr. Price's research time was the multiple roles calcium plays in the functions of the body. These studies virtually forced themselves upon him as medical and dental literature contained such little information about calcium and its important functions.

- A list of calcium functions follows:
  * Every cell is dependent on the presence of ionic calcium.
  * It is used in teeth and bones and the movement of muscles.
  * It is required for the rhythmic action of the heart and the intestines.
  * It is essential for the clotting of blood.
  * It plays a role in infections, pregnancy, and in the maintenance of the acid-alkaline balance.
  * Its presence or absence is a factor in the formation of tooth decay, pyorrhea, and the degenerative diseases.

- The great contributions made by Melvin Page, D.D.S. that have advanced some of the Price findings were discussed; for instance, how routine calcium and phosphorous blood test readings can be used to balance body chemistry. Inasmuch as this is not Price research, I suggest readers go over the chapter again to learn the significance of the Dr. Page contributions to our knowledge of calcium metabolism.

- Dr. Price showed beginning awareness of what Page discovered later when he wrote, "What is important is not so much the presence or absence of an available supply of calcium, such as the calcium in foods, as it is the mechanisms that govern the metabolism of calcium."

- Another great finding was that of the relationship between the thyroid gland's activity and that of the parathyroid.

- The last pages of this chapter listed 16 points involving basic changes that Price found were produced in humans and animals from dental infections. I suggest you turn back a page or so to review his 16 points and the four concluding statements, as each of those statements is a summary of the Price discoveries and their relevance to the prevention of the degenerative diseases.

CHAPTER 12

The Heart and Circulatory System
The Organ Most Often Attacked by Root Canal Bacteria

The technical medical names for a wide number of circulatory ill health problems that can occur as side effects to root canal therapy are endocarditis, myocarditis, pericarditis, heart block, aortitis, angina pectoris, phlebitis, arteriosclerosis, hyper and hypotension, anemia, leukopenia, leukocystosis, lymphopenia, lymphocytosis, bacteremia and glycemia.

There is a tendency to regard diseases that can arise from dental infections as being relatively few in number and variation. The preceding list of circulatory diseases that Dr. Price found could result from a dental infection helps us see the enormity of the problem.

During the time of World War I, it was said that 10 to 11 percent of all deaths in the United States and England were due to heart involvement. At the time, most heart cases involved lesions of heart valves and many doctors believed that streptococcal infections were involved as the cause in 90 percent of such cases.

As recently as 1986, the *Mayo Clinic Health Letter* stated that infective endocarditis that involves the interior lining of the heart's pumping chambers and valves is mainly caused by the germ called streptococcus viridans. *These are the very same family of bacteria that Price found to be most often present in infected teeth.*

In view of the importance of streptococcus and other oral bacteria in the cause of heart disease, and the fact that the number of deaths from this illness has increased since Dr. Price's time from 10 percent to more than 50 percent of all deaths currently, the dental profession must reassess its role in preventing and treating this disorder.

Because these bacteria commonly inhabit the mouth and upper respiratory tract and can be stirred up and introduced into the circulation by routine dental care and even prophylaxis, it is now mandatory for dentists to prescribe antibiotics before and after any dental treatment procedures for patients who have endocarditis in order to prevent a secondary reinfection of their hearts. *However, there is little awareness that root canal fillings, infected tonsils, or remaining tonsil tags can be of even greater danger to heart disease patients.*

Of several cases of endocarditis mentioned, one that described the case of a nine year old girl is heart rending. She had been confined to bed for five of her nine years. A culture taken from the pulps of two of her deciduous (baby) teeth was injected into ear veins of three rabbits and each of them developed acute endocarditis and myocarditis, and one also developed rheumatism. One of the rabbits developed the greatest enlargement of a heart ever seen.

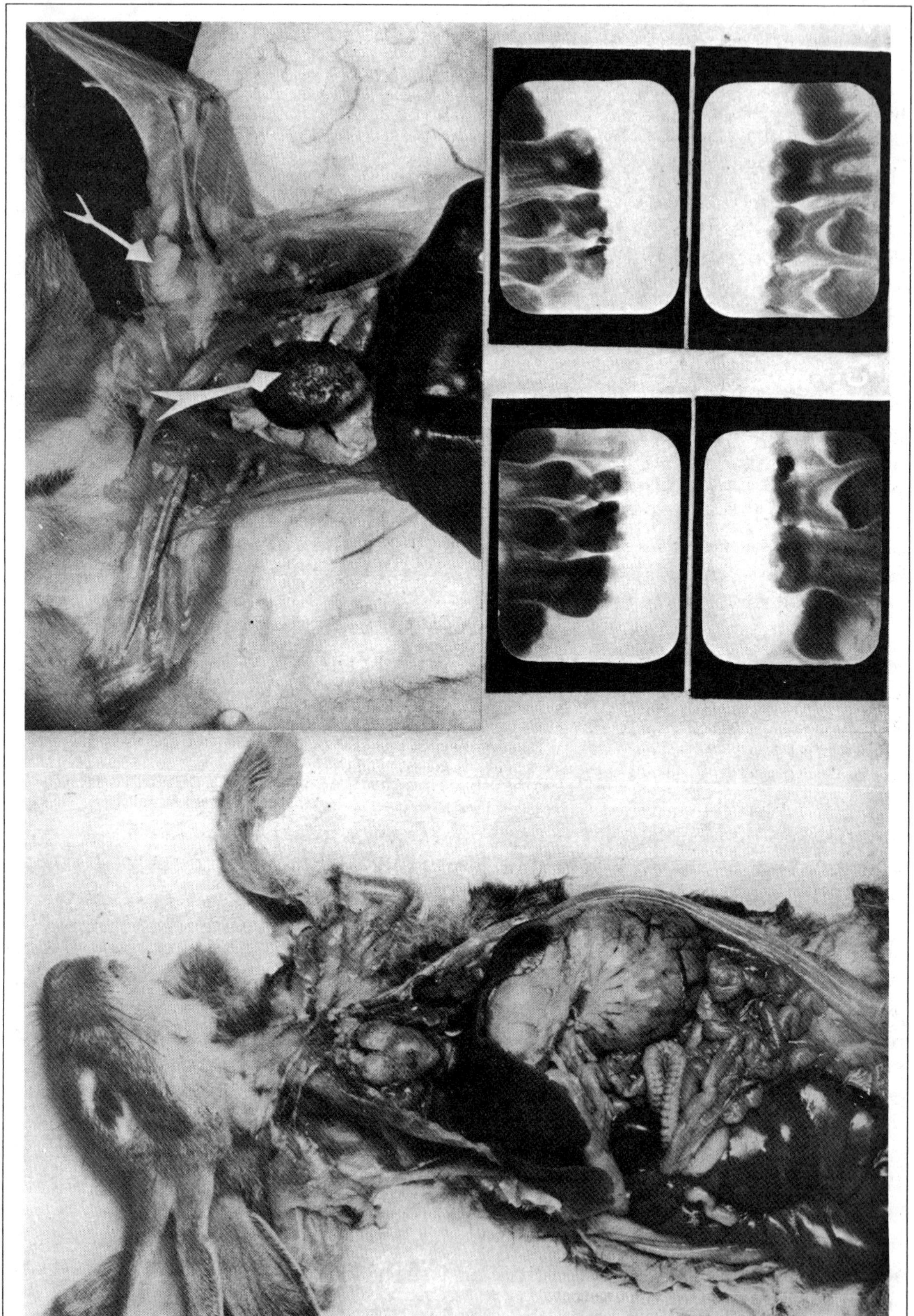

Acute endocarditis in two rabbits from 1 cc. culture from deciduous teeth of a child with endocarditis.

Numbers of children with endocarditis were found to have a delayed loss of their baby teeth due to slow development of the permanent teeth. In addition, a contributing cause was found to be low amounts of ionic calcium in their blood.

Angina pectoris cases exhibited little historical connection to infections. However, several patients with angina, upon removal of infected teeth, had rapid disappearance of their heart pains.

When root filled teeth were removed, many severely affected individuals were able to live a vigorous life again with both comfort and efficiency. A typical case history was a 23 year old woman who was suffering from very acute heart involvement and rheumatism. The heart trouble was so bad that she could hardly walk across the room. After extractions of infected teeth, she gained 15 pounds and for the five years studied while under Dr. Price's care she maintained a perfect health pattern in spite of the fact that both her parents had died of heart involvement between 55 and 60 years of age.

Myocarditis is an inflammation of the muscular walls of the heart. Acute cases are said to have unknown causes. The striking improvement Dr. Price had with these cases made him feel their cause was most often due to the presence of root filled teeth.

Very often in such varied cases it is difficult to classify or generalize about them, as most people have several organs or tissues involved at the same time, and different people display different illnesses. The following is a case of a man who had involvement of many organs:

The patient was 49 years of age and had a complete breakdown in health for some three years. He chiefly complained about his heart. Examination showed it to be enlarged and its apex rotated toward the nipple line. The disturbance had been diagnosed as myocarditis. His blood pressure was up to 180. He complained of extreme tension in his head, and had been diagnosed as having stomach involvement. (See pictures next page)

This patient had undergone several oral examinations as well, and during these appointments he was told that his teeth were fine and that no problems were apparent on his x-ray pictures. However, closer examination revealed putrescent pulps in his first, second, and third molars.

Blood studies showed his ionic calcium was much below normal and blood sugar read 108, non-protein-nitrogen 49, urea 12.5, erythrocytes 5,450,000, polymorphonuclear leucocytes 47.5, and small lymphocytes 47.5 percent.

His facial features were drawn and his actions demonstrated great nervous strain and tension. An anaerobic culture was made from the pulps of the upper left first and second molars. When bacteria from the culture was inoculated into two rabbits, one died in 12 hours with hundreds of small hemorrhages throughout the muscles of the body. The second rabbit's heart had become large and flabby and, when sectioned, profuse hemorrhage in the tissue spaces was discovered.

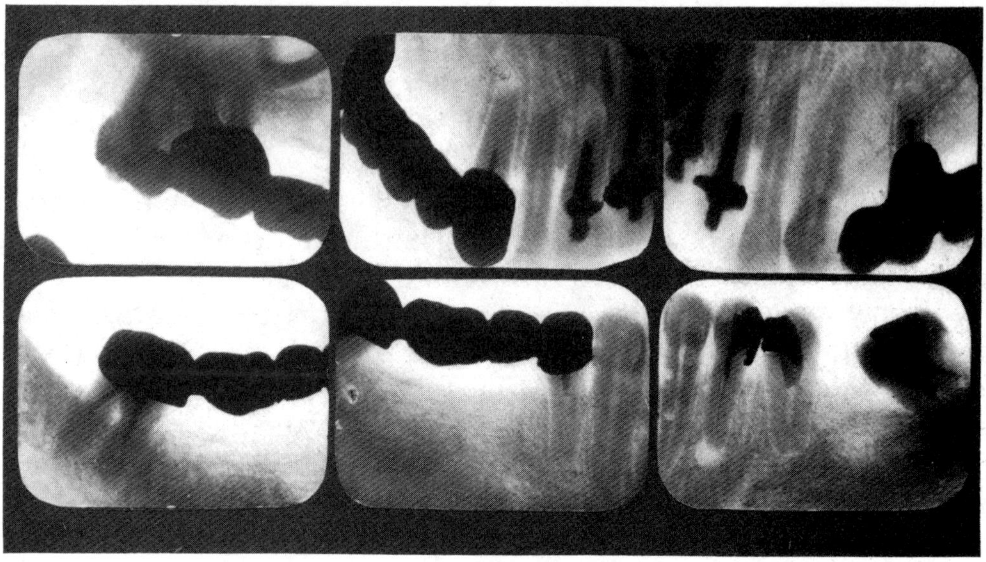

Upper photo: x-ray pictures of dental conditions of patient suffering from severe acidosis, with heart, stomach, and rheumatic involvements.

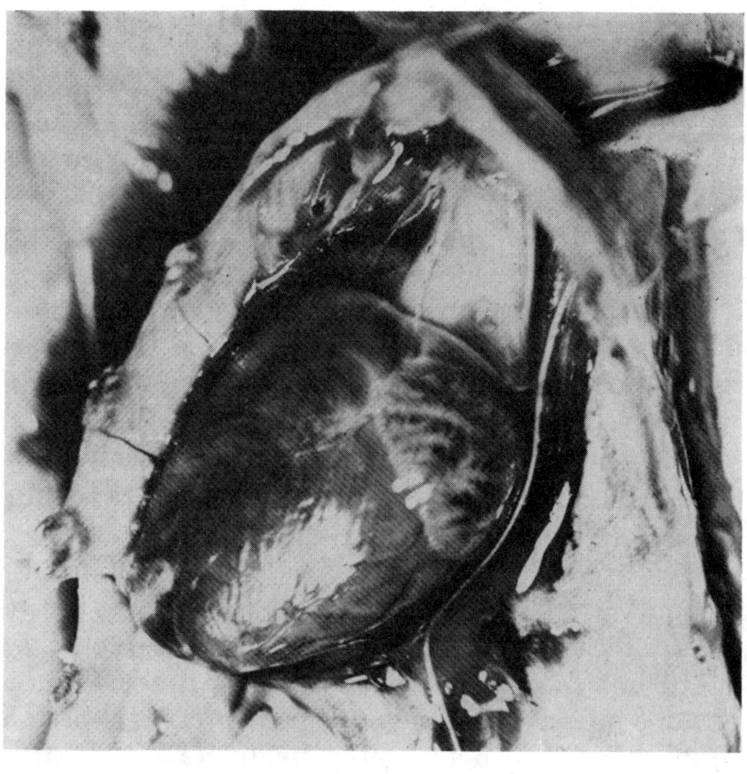

Lower photo: myocarditis with hypertrophy (inflammation and swelling of the heart).

The x-ray pictures of a patient's teeth and heart on page 78 shows an upper left second molar that was extracted and implanted in several rabbits in succession. The first of the five developed hemorrhages and muscle inflammation. The second developed increased amounts of blood in the heart and muscle, muscle atrophy, and edema swelling of the kidney. The third rabbit developed acute appendicitis, minute hemorrhages of the wall of the large intestines, and blood engorgement within the heart muscle and liver. The fourth showed heart and liver atrophy, and the fifth displayed blood engorgement of the heart muscle and kidneys.

The dietary program given the patient may prove of interest. It was a diet rich in calcium, consisting of three to four pints of buttermilk or sweet milk per day, calcium lactate tablets, and parathyroid one-tenth grain daily, later reduced to one-twentieth grain.

A secondary hemorrhage set in after the extraction of the three upper left molars that persisted for hours and required a nurse to be kept in the ward all night. You will remember the inoculated rabbits also developed spontaneous hemorrhages in their muscles.

Further treatment was uneventful. There were no more hemorrhages. In ten days the patient's ionic calcium of the blood was back to normal and the patient stated that he hadn't felt so good in over three years.

Phlebitis cases were few in number so there was some question as to whether dental infections were causative. One phlebitis case that seemed related also displayed a digestive tract disturbance, localizing in the liver and gall bladder. Cultures taken from this woman's root filled tooth and injected into a rabbit showed not only that the bacteria from the tooth caused an acute gall bladder disturbance but that this was accompanied by multiple ulcers — and, in addition, the infection localized in the walls of the rabbit's blood vessels.

An injection made from a culture from the tooth placed in the rabbit's ear caused the ear to swell to the side and to become ten to twenty times the thickness of the other ear. The ear would no longer hold up but dropped to the side, and was very painful to the rabbit when touched. A picture of the rabbit's phlebitis ear appears on the next page.

Many other case histories of patients who had dental infections and heart or other circulatory system involvement were discussed in the two Price volumes. However, the cases mentioned in this chapter give a good cross section of the responses that occurred and how patients improved when bacteria and their toxins were eliminated by the removal of infected teeth.

A good question that may occur to you concerns why a focal infection that has involved an organ or other tissues can heal up and disappear when the infected tooth is extracted. Wouldn't the bacteria in the organ or tissue continue the infection?

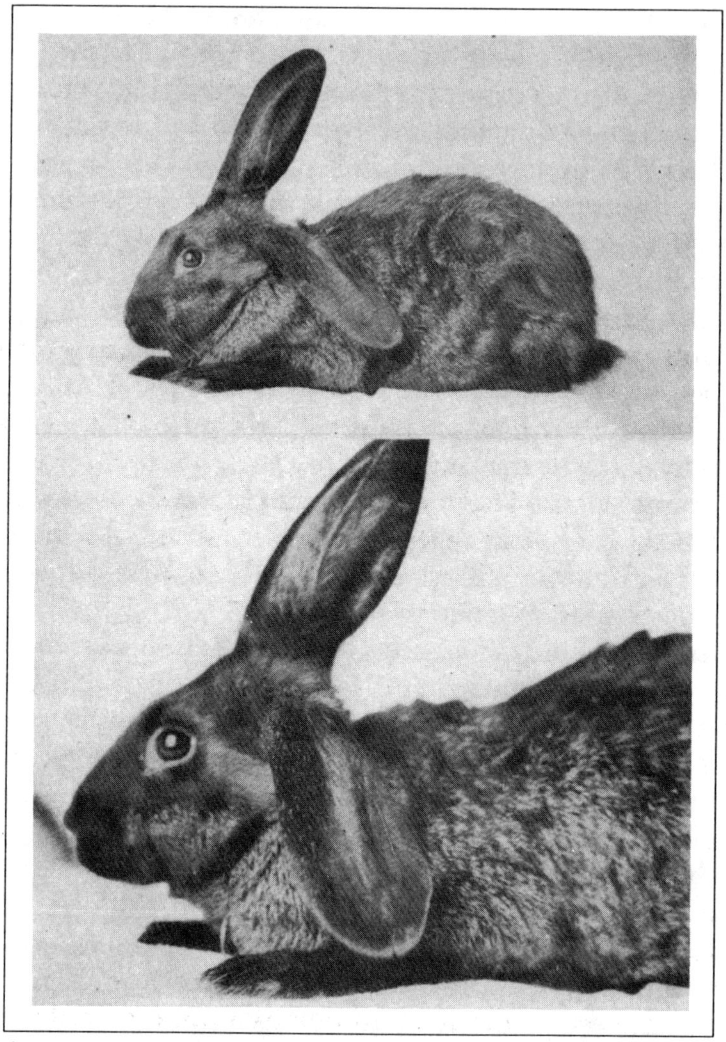

A severe case of phlebitis produced in a rabbit's ear by inoculation with a culture from a tooth of a patient who had recently suffered from a severe phlebitis attack.

The reason healing so often occurs is due to the elimination of the outpouring of bacteria and/or toxins from the tooth as long as it remains present in the mouth. When the tooth is extracted, that infection source is eliminated, giving the immune system a chance to control the bacteria and their toxins and thereby allowing the body to heal itself.

However, if the infection has been causing destructive changes over a protracted period of time, removal of the tooth may not be successful in completely reversing the illness. Even if this is the case, infected tooth removal would at least cut down the possibility of another gland becoming infected, would lessen the tasks confronting the immune system, and would thereby improve the general health status of the patient.

Summary:

- Sixteen heart and other circulatory disease conditions were mentioned as disease problems that can occur as side effects to the presence of root canal filled teeth.

- Such a large number of different heart involvement conditions is surprising as during World War I it was disclosed that 10 to 11 percent of all deaths in the United States and England were due to heart involvement and at that time most cases involved the heart valves.

- During that period most doctors believed these heart cases were caused by streptococcus infections and that this organism species was involved in 90 percent of such cases. The major cause for infective endocarditis accordingto the *Mayo Clinic Health Letter* in 1986 was the streptococcus veridans family of bacteria — the very same one Price found most often arising from infected teeth.

- The number of deaths from heart disease has increased from 10 percent during Price's time to over 50 percent of all deaths today. In view of Price's disclosures about the relationship of root canal therapy to the high number of heart cases and other degenerative diseases related to endodontic treatment, the time is overdue for the dental profession to reassess its role in the occurrence of these diseases.

- A good example of the seriousness of this enquiry can be seen in the endocarditis case of a nine year old girl. She had been bedridden for five of her nine years. A culture made from her two infected baby teeth (see x-ray pictures on inset, page 76) was injected into the ear veins of three rabbits, each of which developed endocarditis and myocarditis, and one of them also developed rheumatism. One of the rabbits developed the largest heart ever seen in a rabbit.

- Numbers of other heart conditions were covered in this chapter. Many of the cases proved difficult to classify as the patients were suffering from several organ or tissue disturbances all at the same time.

- Investigations revealed that in a good number of these cases patients made substantial recoveries when root canal filled teeth were removed.

- Phlebitis cases were few in number but the injection of a culture from a woman patient with phlebitis caused the rabbit's ear to swell 10 to 20 times the thickness that it had been. (See accompanying picture.) In addition, the rabbit developed an acute gall bladder disturbance, multiple ulcers, and infections of the walls of the blood vessels.

- The cases discussed and shown are only a small percentage of heart and circulation cases presented in the two Price books, but they are representative.

- Why these focal infection cases clear up and don't just continue on after the infected tooth or teeth are removed is a question often asked. Undoubtedly, when the condition has persisted for a long period, healing is not fully possible but it is the getting rid of the continual outpouring of bacteria and their toxins from infected teeth that enables the body's immune system to get rid of the infection at the focal infection site and allows the body to heal itself.

CHAPTER 13

It All Starts With a Tiny Cavity; It's a Whole Body Disease, Not a Local One

There have been numerous theories about what actually causes teeth to become decayed. Generally it is agreed that bacteria attach themselves to teeth in the plaque that forms on them from the food we eat. A by-product of the germs that live on teeth is their production of an acid which eats away tooth enamel.

The question is: *Why do some people's teeth develop dental caries and others do not?* Most individuals know that diet has something to do with it — and certainly sugar — but why caries take place remains somewhat mysterious.

It is also common knowledge that tooth decay and the bacteria that accompany it are the forerunners of infection of the tooth's nerve and pulp and the need for root canal treatment.

Dr. Weston Price conducted thousands of experiments to determine the reasons why teeth become carious. Dentists will find that Dr. Price's deductions correspond with current beliefs — but his research brings surprising new insights into the process of tooth decay.

Important basic factors that would have greatly advanced the course of dentistry were buried right along with Price's root canal infection information because of disputes that existed at the time in medicine and dentistry about the focal infection theory.

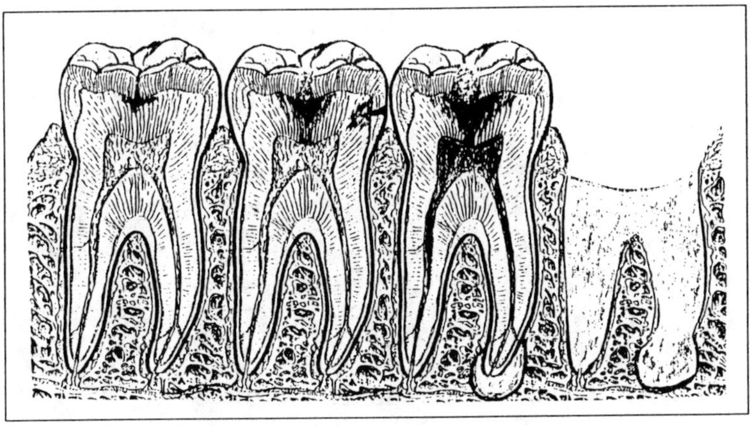

Progress of tooth decay.

Dr. Price made thousands of studies of patients' blood in looking for the true causes of oral diseases. The first key issue he found concerning dental infections was the changing of the acid-base balance of the body from its normal slightly alkaline status to one that was acid.

Studies later by Harold F. Hawkins, D.D.S. showed that the saliva of people who were free of tooth decay was on the alkaline side and those who suffered dental caries had saliva that was decidedly acid. In his book, *Applied Nutrition*, Dr. Hawkins points out that acidity of the saliva results when the diet contains white bread, cereals, cookies, cake, sugar, and similar refined foods.

Starchy grain foods and sweets form that sticky plaque on the surface of teeth that we find so difficult to remove during tooth brushing. This plaque is an ideal food source and home for bacteria that live in our mouths. Their acid by-product etches the enamel and starts the decay process.

The two most fundamental factors in all of life's processes, Price felt, were the changes that take place in the acid-base balance of people who have tooth decay and other dental infections and, secondly, the effect dental infections have on the ionic calcium level of the blood. People who had root canal fillings and those who experienced tooth decay were found to have low amounts of calcium. Both Price and Hawkins independently discovered that those people with normal to high levels of calcium in the blood and saliva enjoyed freedom from dental caries.

The advent of the use of fluorine in water supplies, toothpastes, etc., has, to a great extent, led the public to feel that nutritional factors have been over-emphasized and are of little importance. A quick summary of the chemistry involved with the presence of fluorine in teeth will show that fluorine use isn't all that it is cracked up to be.

In spite of its very hard, dense composition, enamel is a porous structure that can absorb a wide variety of substances present in the saliva. These substances can then travel inside the substance of teeth by means of the fluid flow that takes place in the dentin tubules. It is this fluid flow that also carries nutrients that are responsible for keeping teeth alive and healthy. A low amount of calcium in the blood and saliva no doubt plays a role in the dentin tubules and therefore in the susceptibility of teeth to decay.

The enamel of teeth is composed mostly of calcium carbonate. When a person is subjected to the element fluorine, either from dentifrices or from application directly to the teeth by a dentist or hygienist, it is absorbed directly into the enamel and becomes a part of it.

Fluorine present in water supplies ends up being incorporated into the blood and the saliva. Its presence in the saliva bathes the teeth continually, and fluorine in blood is carried into the inside of teeth by blood vessels that enter at the tip of the roots. From there it is absorbed into the dentin tubules and transported directly into the enamel. Once in the enamel, fluorine combines with the tooth's calcium to form calcium fluoride.

You have been led to believe that fluorine makes teeth harder. The fact is, it actually makes teeth softer. Any dentist who has treated numbers of people who have grown up in areas where the natural water supply is high in fluorine will testify that not only do these people's teeth develop fluorosis, an ugly brownish grey stain throughout their enamel, but when these teeth are drilled they are obviously much softer than the teeth of most of the population. The American Dental Association admits that when fluorine is added to the water supply at the recommended dose of one part per million, ten percent of those using it have some degree of fluorosis.

The reason teeth become softer is because calcium fluoride is not nearly as hard a structure as calcium carbonate. You would think that teeth treated with fluorine would decay much more readily since they are softer. Calcium fluoride, however, is less soluble to attacks by acids than calcium carbonate, so acids created by the bacteria in the plaque are not as successful in etching the enamel and thereby the amount of decay is reduced.

There is a feeling that fluorine treated teeth give protection against caries for a lifetime. Many studies have shown that this protection disappears toward the end of the teenage years.

Because the use of fluorine cuts down the need for dental treatment, it encourages people to believe that it's okay to eat sweets and junk food that is made so readily available.

Probably the most unexpected finding of Dr. Price's investigation was that people who have tooth decay are also more susceptible to degenerative disease afflictions such as those involving rheumatism, tonsils, the heart, neck, internal organs, and nervous system. Diseases of these body areas were grouped together, as all of them are produced by streptococcal infections, the same bacteria involved for the most part in dental diseases.

One can't study about tooth decay without also giving thought to the problems of periodontal disease (pyorrhea). Those who have a marked tendency to develop dental caries are also prone to develop degenerative disease afflictions and, in addition, their ionic calcium level is depressed.

On the other hand, those who aren't susceptible to tooth decay but have a susceptibility to the development of periodontal disease were found, for the most part, *not* to have degenerative diseases — except when periodontal disease became far advanced.

It appears from these factors that dental caries tend to be closely linked to calcium levels of both blood and saliva. Equally important was the discovery that the saliva of patients who have periodontal disease is usually on the alkaline side of neutrality — and that the pus contents in pyorrhea pockets have an even higher alkalinity.

This is of interest, as dentists seldom find teeth decaying in periodontal pockets at the time the disease is active. The softening of the cementum and dentin that sometimes occurs in these areas is often mistaken for caries, but this is a different phenomenon.

All of this information about the various factors involved in the tooth decay process and the differences that exist with periodontal gum problems may seem to have little relevance to the side effects of root canal therapy. However, understanding these basic fundamentals is of utmost importance if the occurrence of these infections inside your teeth are to be prevented.

Other than those teeth that become infected because of injuries, all infections of teeth that require root canal treatment have taken place because the tooth initially had developed tooth decay that extended into the pulp of the tooth, thereby allowing bacteria involved in the decay process to infect its pulp.

Deep pyorrhea pockets can lead to infection inside the tooth when any lateral canals open into the area of the pocket, as this will allow bacteria that are abundant in the pocket to enter these open channels and to travel in them to the pulp and thereby cause it to become infected.

Though the purpose of this book is to reveal the serious possible consequences of infections that reside inside of teeth due to tooth decay and pyorrhea, its dual purpose is to emphasize how brutally urgent is the necessity for people to accept the need for prevention of caries and periodontal problems in the first place.

No longer can we regard the pleasing of our taste buds with sweets and junk food as harmless. Nutritious foods have subtle, delicious tastes that far exceed those sugary, confection-like substitutes presently being consumed in excessive quantities.

Tooth decay can be and is being stopped by diet changes and the side effects are entirely beneficial. Diet improvement leads to a wide variety of health improvements — the most dramatic being the elimination of many degenerative diseases that so plague our society.

With that conclusion to this chapter, I would like to add an additional technical synopsis for dentists reading my compendium. The following is a direct quote of Dr. Price's conclusion to his Chapter 29 dealing with this subject.

Summary and Conclusions

Dental caries are dependent upon the following factors:

(a) A reduction in the hydrogen-ion concentration of the normal environment of the tooth.
(b) An acid producing bacterium.
(c) A change in the chemical constituents of the pabulum bathing the tooth.

All of the above can be modified by proper diet.

Summary:

- To prevent the need for root canal treatments, one must remember that every case needing a root fill, other than those involving injury, started with a tiny bit of tooth decay.

- Why do some people's teeth decay and some do not? That question was central to Price's enquiry.
- Seeing all the diseases that happened to patients resulting from the neglect of tooth decay and to animals when implanted with infected teeth made Dr. Price more and more concerned about the need for cavity prevention.
- Those feelings led him to conduct thousands of blood and saliva experiments on humans and animals that brought forth many insights into the reasons teeth become carious. Unfortunately much of this data was buried right along with his root canal infection discoveries because of disputes over the focal infection theory.
- The two main discoveries regarding the causes of tooth decay were 1) the changing of the acid-base balance of the saliva from its normal alkaline status to one of acidity, and 2) the lowering of the ionic calcium levels in both the blood and the saliva.
- Since Dr. Price's time, these two factors were rediscovered by Harold Hawkins, D.D.S., Melvin Page, D.D.S., Emanuel Cheraskin, M.D., D.M.D. and others.
- Acidity of the saliva and lower calcium values resulting from the ingestion of white flour products, sugar, refined grains, and related products is still not fully understood by the average dentist.
- Unfortunately, the dental and medical professions, in pushing the use of flourine in the prevention of caries, have failed to see that the process of tooth decay is a systemic, whole body problem — not a local one.
- Dentists and physicians have failed to see that systemic health problems are compounded because children and adults who use flourine feel they are protected, and that sweets and refined foods therefore won't hurt their teeth. Furthermore, harmful systemic effects that involve parts of the body other than the mouth are never considered.
- These factors relate to the unexpected findings that people who have tooth decay are also more susceptible to other degenerative diseases.
- A rather high percentage of people whose mouths are overly alkaline tend to develop periodontal disease (pyorrhea). Usually they don't develop tooth decay until the gum disease is far advanced. The softening of the dentin

and cementum in these cases is often mistaken for caries but is a different phenomenon.

- Knowing the chemistry involved in the occurrence of tooth decay and pyorrhea is fundamental to the understanding of these two diseases. When tooth decay is present, the acid-base balance is depressed. That means it is on the acid side and the level of calcium is lower than normal. For those who have pyorrhea, the contents of the pockets are very alkaline and the calcium level is higher than normal.

- Pockets can be the cause of the need for root canal treatment whenever a lateral accessory root canal opens into an infected pocket area, thereby allowing the bacteria in the pocket to be introduced into the tooth through the blood vessels that reside in the root canal.

- Whereas it is hoped that the future will disclose ways for dentists to irradicate infection in dentin tubules, the most important message involved in this book is that every reader must become thoroughly committed to the prevention of tooth decay and periodontal gum infections — thereby dramatically lessening the need for endodontic dental treatment.

CHAPTER 14

X-Ray Pictures Fantastic But Have Limitations

The public and the medical/dental profession alike universally believe that dental x-ray pictures reveal the presence of infection, the extent of it if present, and that from such pictures a treatment plan can be determined.

Yet every dentist knows that there are frequently patients who suffer mild or even severe toothaches that defy detection of infection or pathology through oral examination or x-ray pictures.

Because of the limited amount of room inside the mouth due to the location of the cheekbones, the hard palate, and other facial features, it is — for the most part — impossible to obtain a straight-on x-ray picture of teeth. This results in distortion of the image and a frequent hiding of abnormal changes that may be present. The dental profession has become quite expert at minimizing such problems but difficulties do exist and they must be taken into consideration when assessing whether pathology is present.

In an earlier chapter, I described how lateral accessory root canals can open into the back part of a root and become infected, but not be visible on x-ray pictures. It is also not unusual for a dentist to remove a tooth having an obvious infection at the end of the root and have the patient still complain of a toothache. Further investigation finally discloses the presence of infection of a tooth nearby the one just removed. The picture on the following page shows some of the hidden conditions that can exist.

For this reason people often think their dentist removed the wrong tooth. What has occurred is that the first tooth extracted may or may not have been involved in the cause of the toothache, but it showed more obvious pathology problems and it did need removal. The continued pain reveals the fact that a second tooth is involved. This happens more often than one might imagine.

Cracks in teeth from injuries or biting on something hard can also be difficult to locate and are almost never visible on x-ray pictures. It is such frequent circumstances and frustrations that keep the life of a dentist far from being dull.

Dentists are taught to tell patients to have any root canal fillings they have checked every year or two, as we know that no matter how excellent the treatment, hidden lateral canals that cannot be seen on x-ray pictures can contain infection. Patients invariably forget this advice and, because of the desire to limit the use of radiation, they and their dentist often put off these follow-ups. As we discussed, even when teeth appear perfectly normal on examination and on x-ray pictures, Price found thousands of cases that still contained bacteria and their toxins.

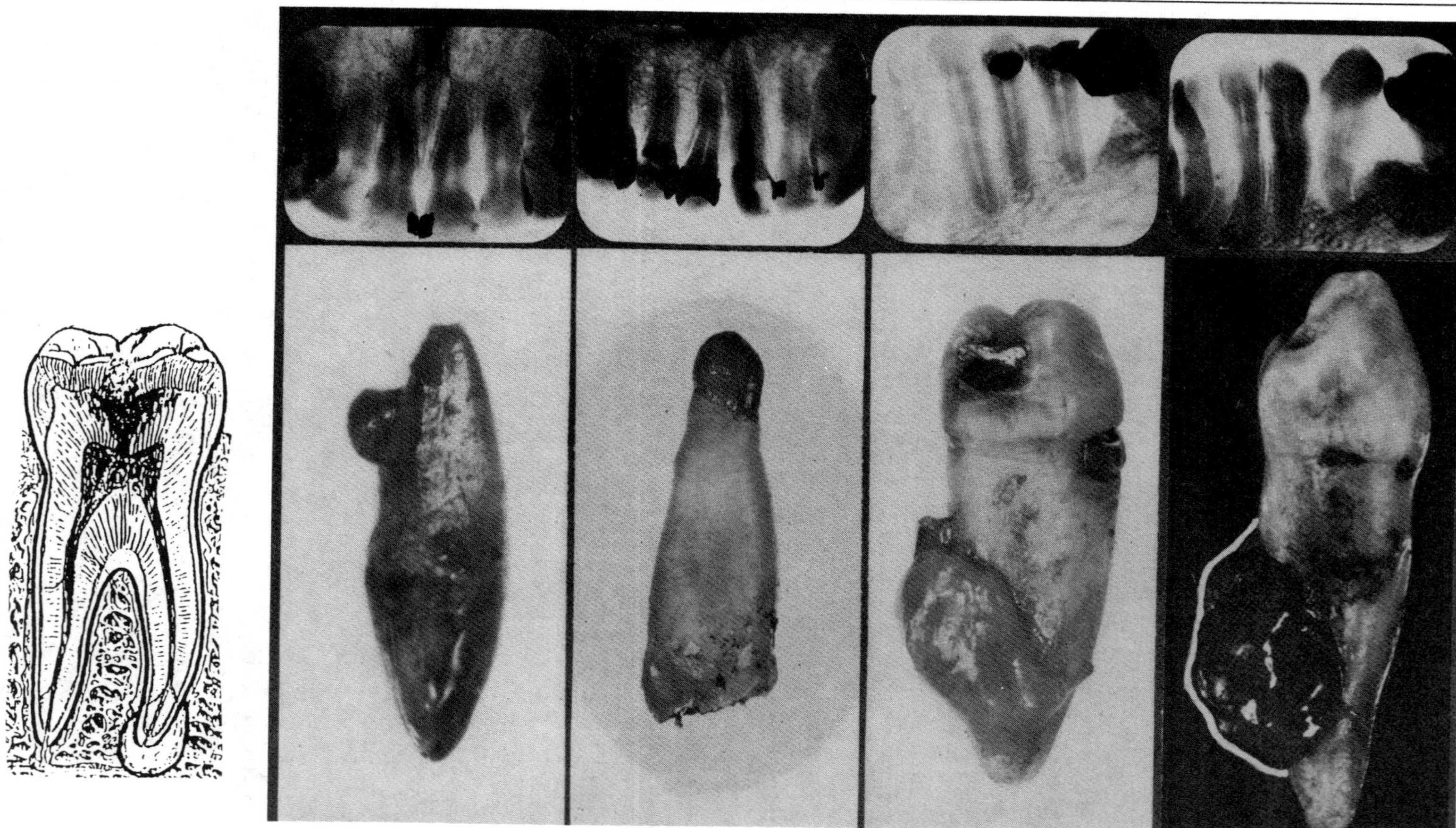

Comparison of the roentgenographic and photographic appearances of extracted teeth when they are rotated, allowing the infected area to be seen. Molar tooth showing progress of decay in enamel; dentin exposing the pulp. Bacteria in pulp causing its death, and a granula at the end of the root.

It is common and logical to assume that when a large area of destruction appears in the bone at the end of the root of a tooth, a severe dental infection is present. However, as was previously stated, Dr. Price discovered that the bacterial count and severity of infection was often much worse in those having only small amounts of bone loss around the root ends of teeth than those exhibiting a greater degree of bone destruction. Of course, both of these are bad situations to have present in one's mouth, but the difference in the bacterial activity of each discloses how much misunderstanding exists concerning the infections of teeth.

Most dentists today, I dare say, will find the information presented in the previous paragraph unbelievable. To sceptics, may I refer you to an article that appeared in *Oral Surgery*, 1966; 21; 659 by Dr. S.N. Baskar, and another by M.H. Stern that appeared in the *Journal of Dental Research*, 1979; 50; 130.

Both pointed out that the visual areas of abnormalities on x-ray pictures are not necessarily areas of infecton harboring bacteria. Dr. Stern stated that, for the most part, *such visible areas are lesions that have been identified as radicular cysts and granulomas. The granulomas are reactive lesions caused by bacterial destruction originating from an infected root canal that opens into that area. Experiments indicate that the granuloma is a response of cells to the bacteria in the root canal but, at the same time, bacterial cultures taken from the areas of lost bone at the root end of the tooth have proven negative 85 to 100 percent of the time.*

These studies are yet another substantiation of discoveries made by Dr. Price in this regard some 45 years previous to the publication of the Baskar and Stern articles.

There are numerous other types of pathologic conditions that challenge the diagnostic ability of dentists. Some of these conditions are misinterpreted as tooth infections, but as descriptions of them would require complicated explanations that are not germane to the purposes of this book, I mention them only to further indicate the number of difficulties inherent in the use of dental x-ray pictures in the interpretation of dental pathology.

These statements in no way imply that the use of x-ray examinations are not of tremendous help. They are presented so the public can better understand the complexities involved in dealing with oral infections and why, at times, what is seen on an x-ray picture may not be what it seems to be. The beauty of Price's work is the clarification it brings to the confusion and misinterpretation that exists.

Summary:

- The formation of the hard palate, cheekbones, narrowness of jaws and positions of teeth make the taking of accurate x-ray pictures a challenge.

- For these reasons x-ray pictures of teeth and jaws quite often fail to disclose the presence of infection or what kind of treatment might be required, contrary to the generally accepted views of most dentists and patients.

- Cracks in teeth are almost never visible on x-ray pictures.

- The extent of bone loss around a tooth, though felt to indicate the severity of its infection, does not do so. Doctors Baskar and Stern, in separate studies, reported that 85 to 100 percent of dental granulomas and radicular cysts do not contain bacteria. This does not mean the tooth itself is not infected.

- When the dentist removes or treats a tooth but the patient continues to have a toothache, it may seem that the wrong tooth was removed. The pictures in this chapter show how a second tooth is often involved.

- Because lateral canals can contain infection, dentists have been taught to advise that root filled teeth be re-x-rayed each year or two.

- None of this infers that the use of x-ray pictures is to no avail. Quite the contrary, good x-ray pictures often disclose disease conditions that should receive immediate attention if the patient's health is not to be jeopardized.

CHAPTER 15

How the Immune System Becomes Overloaded

When isn't it a good time to undergo root canal treatment?

Dr. Price didn't say it was never appropriate to undergo root canal therapy. However, let me quote a short paragraph of his that introduces stress factors that can overload the immune system.

Contributing Overloads Which Modify Defensive Factors: What are the contributing factors causing a break in resistance?

> *"Dental infections, while potentially harmful, may not be causing apparent or serious injury until the individual is subjected to some other overload, at which time a serious break may come. The chief contributing overloads are influenza, pregnancy, lactation, malnutrition, exposure, grief, worry, fear, heredity, and age."*

Careful analysis of large numbers of cases at several different time intervals demonstrated that a high percentage of people experiencing such stressors developed what Dr. Price called "rheumatic degenerative group lesions." Such cases involved rheumatism of the joints and muscles, the heart, nerve tissues, kidneys, and the digestive tract, including the appendix. Because tuberculosis and pneumonia often have streptococcal involvement, they too should be considered.

INFLUENZA—THE FLU

The two foremost stress factors that Dr. Price felt were compromised by the presence of root canal fillings were the FLU and PREGNANCY.

During the flu epidemic of 1918, Dr. Price studied 260 influenza patients in five different hospitals. This study was exceedingly difficult because so many were so seriously ill that questioning and x-ray examinations were often not possible. Patients were divided into two groups: those having dental infections, and those free from oral problems.

Realizing that under the circumstances numbers of infected teeth must have been missed, the percentage of individuals developing serious complications, including pneumonia, emphysema, carditis, severe neuritis, and severe rheumatism, who also had dental infections, numbered around 72 percent. While the percentage of those seemingly free of oral problems but who developed such serious illnesses was only 32 percent.

Another observation, since confirmed by other dentists, was that individuals who had dental infections were more prone to develop the flu than those who kept their mouths in good condition.

In another test, washings from the nasopharynges of flu patients were inoculated into the throats of rabbits, resulting in the development of pneumonia in the rabbits. When a culture from a root filled tooth was added to the throat inoculation, the rabbit developed streptococcal pneumonia.

Statistics accumulated in England and Wales two years after the flu epidemic showed that approximately four times as many died from complication illnesses as did from the flu attack itself.

Dr. Price's studies showed that the occurrence of complicating illnesses was two and one-third greater in those individuals having dental infections as in the group free from dental infections.

During the course of illness, patients with and without dental infection often suffer from depression and exhaustion. However, those without dental infection often readily recover, while those with a focal infection find themselves a victim of something they cannot recognize that often results in some gland or tissue becoming a new source of illness. Bacteria, as they travel around the body in the bloodstream, have an uncanny ability to select the weakest body part as an ideal place to set up a second residence.

PREGNANCY—LACTATION

Among those we considered not susceptible to illness, the percentage of men and women is quite evenly divided. As susceptibility increases, this changes from 50-50 to 93 percent of females having strong inheritance factors and only seven percent for males. Dr. Price's studies indicate that the most important factors accounting for why these figures so drastically change are the stresses involved in motherhood and lactation.

Certainly physical injuries, extreme anxiety, exposure, nutrition, hunger, exhaustion, acute and chronic infections, alcohol, and drugs all contribute singly or collectively to break a person's otherwise well-working immune system. The presence of focal infection, as we have seen, compounds and magnifies every facet of ill health.

Dr. Price found that many new and expectant mothers developed acute rheumatism during the period of gestation or lactation. A typical case is that of a young woman of 22 years who had a physique and physical reserve well above average. She decided to undertake the responsibilities of motherhood, and the birth of a baby that was unusually robust followed.

During the early period of breastfeeding, the young mother developed such severe rheumatism that she could not take care of herself or her baby. However, a couple of infected teeth were removed and she immediately improved. Though her relief was not complete, she continued nursing her

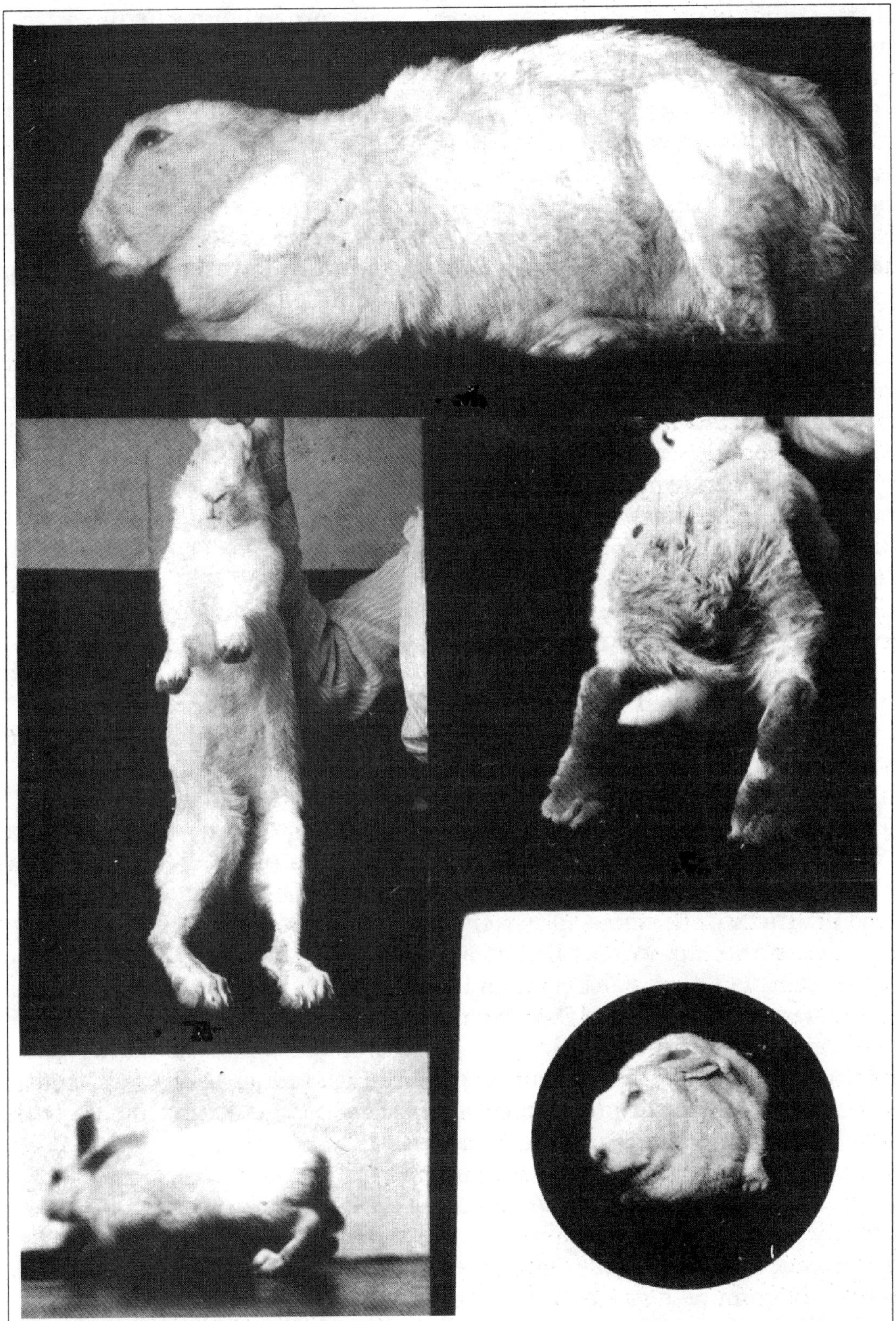

Various views of a rabbit paralyzed by an inoculation of infected dental culture from a woman with a pregnancy overload.

child for about six months. Thereafter her remaining rheumatism disappeared. During the lactation period, she had been drinking large quantities of milk; this could have helped her calcium levels, but we now know that a high milk intake depletes magnesium. It was later found that in childhood this young woman had suffered mild endocarditis which left a mitral valve leakage.

Because this clinical picture of a weakened immune system being more susceptible to the health hazards of infections in teeth was repeatedly demonstrated, a further test on a rabbit was undertaken. The rabbit they selected had recovered from a condition of complete paralysis of the first vertebra with loss of continence of urine and feces, plus loss of all motor and sensory control of its back legs. This rabbit had recovered so completely as to appear normal. The only reminder of its previous severe condition was a slight rotation of its one hind leg.

The ability of this rabbit's immune system to overcome a root canal infection inoculation was tested by mating it with a male rabbit. At the beginning of pregnancy, the rabbit appeared to be in very good physical condition; it was fat, its coat sleek, and in every way she seemed a normal, healthy rabbit.

The inoculation had caused no visible ill health effects throughout the pregnancy period. Five young were born which, at birth, seemed to have developed normally. However, these baby rabbits all died in a few hours to one and one-half days after birth. It became apparent that the inoculated disease stress overload left the mother rabbit without the ability to produce milk and feed her young.

A few days after the birth, this rabbit became nervous, began losing weight, and developed a marked disturbance of her central nervous system. The least excitement would cause her to fall over on her side. She eventually developed pneumonia and died in about five weeks.

Upon culturing the bacteria in her lungs, the research team found streptococcus and diplococcus bacteria similar to those that were present in the tooth that had been cultured and inoculated under the skin.

It was Dr. Price's opinion that though her spine had healed from the original paralyzing infection, the organisms were retained but controlled. This rabbit had built up protection and immunity but the overload stress of the pregnancy and lactation, *combined with the tooth infection*, caused the original infection to again become rampant.

TRAUMA—INJURY

When people suffer a severe auto accident, fall, or suffer some other injury, their immune system is called upon to work at peak performance in order for the patient to achieve a speedy recovery. Those people with root canal fillings are generally found to have a healing rate slower than expected. Quite often, the extra stress that the injury places on their defense system allows the organisms to get out of hand and attack some other organ or tissue.

We all know of individuals who get over one illness only to develop another. This can, of course, happen when no dental infections or root canals are present because of poor nutrition, anxiety, alcohol and drug use, and a whole variety or combination of other stresses with which humans must cope. The more stress involved, the more the immune system is taxed to keep the person alive and functioning.

When the body is continually subjected to irritation in any one or a number of its tissues and parts, these areas often become sick. Take Dr. Price's story of the man who came to America by ship in steerage from the Philippines to San Francisco and from there by train to Cleveland. All during the travel time, he was confined to relatively small areas where exercise was impossible and movement was restricted.

In Cleveland he worked as a night watchman in a manufacturing plant. It was necessary for him to walk several miles each night over acres of cement floors. Because he didn't wear rubber heels on his shoes, the irritation to his knee joints and ankles was stressful and made him uncomfortable.

After a few weeks he developed acute rheumatism in the joint areas. At that point, an oral examination disclosed some dental infections. The sources of infection were removed and with the addition of rubber heels to his shoes, his problems were relieved and he was able to continue the same occupation with no further symptoms of rheumatism.

Dr. Price also relates the case of a patient who suffered eye problems and was unable to read for any length of time without periods of rest. This had been a continuing problem for several years and glasses proved to be of no help. After removal of dental infections, this patient was able to discard the glasses he had worn for 15 years, and reading for long periods no longer caused discomfort.

Many other patients who wore glasses reported such improvement of their eyes after the removal of dental infections that their eye glass prescriptions had to be reduced, and others were able to discontinue using glasses altogether.

I must report here that Dr. Melvin Page in St. Petersberg Beach, Florida, found that infected tonsils, and tags left from incomplete removal of tonsils, were a common source of focal infection quite equal to dental infections in their severity and ability to cause diseases to occur in other body tissues.

GRIEF and WORRY

We all know of individuals that were so grief stricken at the death of a loved one that they also died a short time later. Just a year ago, I experienced such a situation. Two wealthy, spinster neighbors were inseparable. All that knew them felt it would be tragic for the survivor when one of them died. A year ago one did die and the other passed away just three days later.

Dr. Price reported a family of five girls who nursed their father through a long illness until his death of pernicious anemia. His problems had followed the death of the mother from a heart condition.

These girls were not physically exhausted by their duties to their father because with five of them they were able to spread the work load among them. However, each one developed rheumatic group lesions. One neuritis, two developed heart trouble, and two rheumatism. Oral examinations disclosed that all had infected teeth; removal relieved their illnesses. The stress to their immune systems was such that it could no longer cope with the bacteria hiding in their teeth.

EXPOSURE

It is common to hear someone say that due to a cold winter wind or draft they became ill. Another might get a stiff neck or shoulder from exposure to cold.

Dr. Price reported the case of a man who was having infected teeth treated. The man was working in a factory when a water main line burst. In order to prevent damage to the factory, he worked outside in the cold of winter in icy water for two hours repairing the break.

He had been receiving dental treatment because of his neuritis and after this incident his condition became so bad that his knees were drawn up to his chin for many weeks and one arm was almost useless from atrophy.

To test the ability of exposure to cold to cause illness, cultures were made from the teeth of a patient suffering rheumatism. Inoculations were made of these bacteria into four rabbits. Two were kept in a warm cage and the other two had their hind legs immersed in water with ice in it. The dosages in these cases were purposely kept small. All four rabbits received 12 inoculations at the same time over a 32 day period.

All of the rabbits lost weight following the inoculations. The two control rabbits in warm cages lost 10 percent of their weight, while the two exposed to ice water lost 14 percent. The weight changes proved to be the least important finding.

The two control rabbits that were not exposed to chilling did not develop any lesions from the inoculations. Both gained weight. One was still alive four months later and was so healthy that it was used for another experiment subsequently.

However, the two exposed to chilling developed severe rheumatic lesions. One developed abscesses of the left shoulder extending into the muscle. The other rabbit developed arthritis of the right shoulder and left leg joint, which is comparable to our wrist.

The rabbits' response to cold illustrates how humans also react, especially when there is any type of infection present. We also experience weight loss, stiff joints, rheumatism, etc. Inasmuch as the researchers found ionic calcium values reduced in those with dental infections, it is easy to see how exposure to cold could cause a further reduction of calcium that would be instrumental in the occurrence of ill health symptoms.

Treatment that included the elimination of any body infections, applications of heat, massage, and the addition of a calcium supplement proved successful in cases related to exposure to cold. Incidentally, experiments using massage on humans and animals showed that increases of calcium occurred in their blood.

NUTRITION and HUNGER

Any machine we use is dependent upon fuel to operate. Likewise, well-being is dependent on the nature, quantity, and quality of the foods people consume. However, it is increasingly clear that the average person thinks that whatever is put into the body through the mouth will adequately feed the body.

Studies after World War I of North Carolina mountaineers found their diets to be largely fat pork, coffee, and grits made of white corn, combined with a liberal use of tobacco, chiefly snuff. Sometime later, studies made in the southern states of Georgia, Alabama, Louisiana, Arkansas and Texas showed that people were living on equally deficient diets. These individuals for the most part were underweight, nervous, irritable, and old-appearing at relatively young ages. Such poor dietary conditions still exist in a number of areas today.

The most striking finding in such studies was the prevalence of serious degenerative diseases. Many homes had one or more bedridden with endocarditis, acute rheumatism, chronic arthritis, and a number suffered digestive and nervous system disorders — not to mention a high degree of tooth decay and pyorrhea.

It has been demonstrated by a number of scientists that deficient diets result in the same diseases as are caused by infections. Dr. Price also made extensive studies of the reactions of animals inoculated with different strains of dental infection bacteria, and these repeatedly produced symptoms and lesions which resemble — to a marked degree — those that are produced by deficient diets.

Studies demonstrated that the immune systems of animals on deficient diets led to more advanced systemic pathologic diseases and, conversely, those on good diets responded less quickly to the onslaught of the introduction of dental infections and had better survival rates.

That being stated, it should be said that during Price's studies it was found that many animals on deficient diets still had a remarkable power of defense against infection, though not equal to those on normal diets. A particular problem of deficient diets was the production of low ionic calcium which, in turn, lowered the animals' defense to dental infections.

OTHER OVERLOAD STRESSES THAT INCREASE SUSCEPTIBILITY

Physical and nervous exhaustion, when it exists for prolonged periods, increases one's susceptibility and reaction to dental infections. Likewise, no one will dispute that the presence of other types of acute or chronic infections such as diphtheria, salmonella infections, candidiasis, syphilis, and other sexual diseases accentuate the severity of reactions from oral infections.

Alcohol and other drugs are well-known as substances that increase pathologic effects, including those that arise from dental infections and their toxins. Price's studies revealed that alcoholics are more susceptible to streptococcal infection from focal infection sources.

Many people have expressed appreciation of the dental profession and the high interest dentists have demonstrated over many, many years of encouraging the public to adopt preventive dentistry principles and better nutrition in order to save their teeth and reduce the need for dental treatment.

Those who neglect such preventive advice, not only find that their oral diseases become more extensive, but also that the additional dental services they require make their dental treatment needs much more costly. The prevention of the need for root canal treatment by the early discovery of the presence of tooth decay is a prime example.

Poor diet practices create vitamin and mineral starvation that, in turn, produces overload stress similar to that caused by disease. In addition, deficient diets, particularly those resulting in upset calcium balances, tend to directly lower the body's defense against dental infections and can severely alter other metabolic functions.

Throughout my life, I have been vitally interested in how the body functions and the effects of nutrition on health. To this has now been added the related avocation of informing the public about the relative safety that can be theirs when they avoid the need for root canal therapy by adopting good nutritional habits and by seeing their dentist two to three times per year for regular and thorough prophylaxis and examination. The consequent positive overall health effects of such preventive practices are what everyone hopes to achieve.

Summary:

- What factors contribute to an overload of the immune system that cause a previously healthy person to become ill?

- If a person's root canal filling has not been affecting their health, what happens to change that status?

- Dr. Price pointed out that sudden overloads or changes such as the flu, a severe accident, pregnancy, breastfeeding, malnutrition, excessive worry, grief, and age could tax the efforts of the immune system to such an extent that it could no longer control the bacteria and toxins coming from the root filled tooth or teeth.

- Influenza: During the flu epidemic of 1918, Price studied 260 influenza patients in five different hospitals. He studied both those who had dental infections and those free of infections.

- Those who developed complications such as pneumonia, emphysema, carditis, severe neuritis, and severe rheumatism and also had dental infections numbered 72 percent. Those free of dental problems who developed such illnesses were only 32 percent.

- Those who were free of dental infections were not apt to get the flu in the first place.

- Rabbits inoculated with nasal washings of patients with dental infections developed pneumonia.

- Statistics from England published two years after the flu epidemic disclosed that four times as many people died of complications than from the flu itself.

- Pregnancy and lactation: Men and women as a group are evenly divided in their susceptibility to illness. That percentage increases to 93 percent of females and only 7 percent of males because of inheritance factors. The most important factors accounting for this change proved to be pregnancy and lactation.

- New and expectant mothers having infected teeth frequently developed acute rheumatism. Inoculations from such patients into rabbits produced multiple illnesses in the rabbits.

- Injury: Those who suffered accidents or injuries and had mouth infections were generally found to have slower than expected healing rates. We all know people who no more get over one illness when they get another.

- Grief: We all know of people so grief stricken at the loss of a loved one that they develop a series of illnesses and/or die a short time later.

- Exposure: Whenever I heard of a person contracting a cold or a stiff neck from exposure to the cold, I was somewhat skeptical until I read of a Price research project on the subject.

- Inoculations were made from a patient with rheumatism into four rabbits. Two were kept in warm cages while the other two had their hind legs immersed in ice water. These two developed rheumatic lesions, plus one developed an abscess in the left shoulder and the other arthritis of the right shoulder and leg joint. The two in the warm cage remained in good health.

- Nutrition: Contrary to our experience with humans, animals on deficient diets were often found by Dr. Price to have an outstanding ability to ward off infections. This ability was lost with aging.

- Animals on good diets were somewhat slower to develop degenerative diseases when challenged with root canal inoculations than those on poor diets.

- Most interestingly, the reactions of animals to dental infection bacteria often produced lesions that were remarkably like those produced by humans on deficient diets.

- People living in remote areas of North Carolina, Arkansas and Texas living on fat pork, corn grits, coffee and tobacco were generally underweight, nervous, irritable, old appearing at young ages, prone to nutritional deficiency diseases, and easy prey to numbers of illnesses.

- The average dentist regularly goes out of his way to teach patients how to prevent dental problems from occurring, thereby diminishing the need for their services. In effect, we are one of the only business or profession continually striving to minimize our business!

CHAPTER 16

It Isn't Only the Bacteria from Root Canal Filled Teeth That Cause These Diseases in Rabbits — Does the Amount of Infection Influence the Severity of the Disease?

We are all aware that organisms that produce disease vary greatly in the amount and severity of their virulence. Because teeth are relatively small, it is also generally believed that when a tooth has a properly treated root canal filling, it is impossible for an infection therefrom to overwhelm the patient. Furthermore, many express the opinion that the organisms which cause dental infections are low in virulence and that the occurrence of any systemic involvement is unlikely or, at best, of minor significance.

One of the first of numerous experiments by Dr. Price was to withdraw the moisture content of an extracted tooth in a drying chamber. Measuring the amount of dehydration showed that roughly five percent of the volume of every root filled tooth is a fluid which can quite readily become a culture medium that can become easily saturated with abundant bacteria.

In another experiment, a root filled tooth was taken from a patient suffering acute endocarditis. The tooth was crushed and the particles washed. The settled wash liquid was then injected into a rabbit. The weight of the organisms injected was determined by counting the number present in the dilution; the actual amount the rabbit received was only a millionth part of a gram. Still, the rabbit became seriously ill with endocarditis. With such a small amount of bacteria involved, the question arose as to whether something more than the bacteria could be the causative agent.

To answer this question, the same crushing and washing of extracted root filled teeth was undertaken but then the liquid was centrifuged, thereby removing the bacteria. Now the one cubic centimeter remaining of bacteria free water-like appearing liquid was injected into rabbits and they too developed heart lesions, even more severely than did rabbits injected with bacteria cultures alone.

In summarizing this particular research data, Dr. Price clarified what transpired:

> *"When infected teeth produce disturbance in other parts of the body, it is not necessary that the quantity of infection be large, nor is it demonstrated that it is necessary that organisms pass throughout the body or to the special tissues involved, but the evidence at hand strongly suggests that soluble poisons may pass from the infected*

teeth to the lymph or blood circulation, or both, and produce systemic disturbance entirely out of proportion to the quantity of poison involved. The evidence indicates that this toxic substance may under certain circumstances sensitize the body or special tissues so that very small quantities of the organisms, which produce that toxin, may produce very marked reactions and disturbances."

In a similar study, instead of testing the effects of root canal filled teeth, an investigation was made of teeth that had pulp or root end infections but had never had root canal treatments. Here again the concern was whether the infection material in teeth had any other contents that were injurious other than microorganisms.

This was an important undertaking because no past records of any studies could be found showing that teeth may contain any injurious substances other than bacteria. Large numbers of studies were made by Dr. Price and others of the organisms that are present or developed in infected teeth. These investigations concerned the identifying of organisms present, their normal biologic properties, and their disease or pathologic producing possibilities.

These procedures involved securing the bacteria found in infected teeth; culturing them in suitable growth media; testing their reactions on various sugars and on animals; and, in addition, determining the character of their structure.

In this way, starting with but a few organisms, large numbers could be grown and produced — thus enabling them to be tested in numerous ways, such as: determining their ability to adjust to new environments, their ability to be transferred to animals for further study, and to test the efficacy of drugs and medications upon their activities.

In this connection one of the Dr. Price studies concerned two rabbits that were full brothers and weighed within an ounce or so of each other. They were kept continually in the same environment after birth and were fed the same diet.

Freshly extracted infected teeth that had not received endodontic treatment were finely crushed and washed, and the washings centrifuged to throw off any sediment and bacteria. One cubic centimeter of the clear, supernatant liquid was injected into rabbit A. Rabbit B, its brother, was the control animal.

Rabbit B continued to gain weight while A slowly began to lose weight, though it had no loss of appetite. Both ate heartily and exercised freely in a roomy cage week after week. Rabbit A kept losing and rabbit B kept gaining weight.

At the end of four weeks, A had lost 25 percent of its original weight and B had gained 10 percent. At the end of the fifth week, rabbit A died, having by then lost 37 percent of its weight. Autopsy studies showed a withering away of its tissues with marked atrophy of all muscle tissue, along with changes to its digestive tract.

In other studies, the Price group found that when organisms were washed free from their culture media and were injected into animals, the animals died in seven days on average, with a loss of weight of two percent per day. When the whole culture was injected, they had a loss of weight of three percent and died within six days. This suggested a toxic factor was present.

In determining the nature of the toxic products, 17 rabbits were injected with filtered washings containing only the toxic substances of the infected teeth. Of these, 13 had a weight loss of 3.8 percent per day and died within 5 days.

Conversely, of 14 rabbits injected with unfiltered washings, on average 8 died in 12 days while suffering a weight loss of 1.8 grams. The researchers were at a loss as to why the toxic substances alone were more rapidly lethal than the toxic substances plus the organisms. Finally they reasoned that the presence of dead or living organisms in the bloodstream or body fluids might call forth antitoxins in the body to combat the invaders.

In view of the fact that it was believed that the only injurious substance in infected teeth were bacteria, Price concluded that:

> *"Infected teeth may contain, in addition to microorganisms, toxic substances which produce very profound effects upon experimental animals and which tend to prepare the tissues of the host, at least in some cases, for a more ready invasion by the organisms growing in that tooth."*

Summary:

- The nature and results of the numerous Dr. Price investigations are a continuous source of amazement.
- For example, in pondering how bacteria could survive in dentin tubules when they become sealed off by the root canal filling, Dr. Price devised a method of dehydrating teeth — that is, measuring the amount of moisture they contain.
- In doing this experiment, Dr. Price found root filled teeth contained fluid that was of sufficient quantity to be a culture medium that would nourish bacteria.

- Another question that interested Dr. Price was whether bacteria that infected teeth contained were solely responsible for the illnesses that occurred to rabbits after infected teeth were imbedded under their skins.

- He found that by extracting infected teeth, crushing them, and then washing the powder, that bacteria could still be found in the liquid. When he put that liquid in a centrifuge, the centrifugal force spun off the bacteria and sediment, leaving a clear liquid.

- When Dr. Price injected a small amount of this clear liquid into a rabbit, it lost 25 percent of its weight in four weeks and it died in the fifth week. Its brother rabbit, used as the control animal and not injected, continued to thrive and gain weight.

- This demonstrated that there were toxins present in this bacteria free liquid lethal enough to kill rabbits. Not only that, when the liquid containing bacteria before it was centrifuged was injected into rabbits, they too lost weight but lived on for 12 days, while those injected with the clear liquid that contained no bacteria survived for only five days.

- This indicated that the toxins were more lethal than the bacteria and the toxins together. Though puzzled by this discovery, the researchers reasoned that when organisms were present, they stimulated the body to form antitoxins that would, for a while, combat the invaders.

- In still another study, the number of organisms were minimized so that only one millionth part of a gram was injected. Still, that small amount taken from an endocarditis heart patient and injected into a rabbit caused the animal to develop endocarditis and die.

- Infective material produced symptoms way out of proportion to the amount injected.

- All of these determinations were original discoveries by Dr. Price. A search of scientific literature revealed no previous studies or investigations on this subject.

CHAPTER 17

Why This Research was Covered-up and Buried
How Focal Infection Theory Disbelievers Brought on This Blunder

How could scientific discoveries as important as these be so completely suppressed? Two or three factors were mainly responsible.

First, all during the time of the Price research there was an intense disagreement among members of both the medical and dental professions as to whether or not the focal infection theory was valid.

As was stated before, this theory contends that infected teeth, tonsils, tonsil tags, and similar other areas that are infected could be responsible for setting up a whole new infection in another tissue or organ of the body because the bacteria involved are transported to the new area via the bloodstream. The views, both pro and con, were fiercely debated and resulted in professional wars — that is, wars between physicians and their medical societies; between dentists and dental societies; between physicians and dentists; and between dentists and physicians. The arguments of believers and non-believers were hot and heavy. These arguments against the acceptance of the theory created a milieu that was not readily receptive to Dr. Price's research results.

Acceptance today of focal infection is so taken for granted that hardly anyone pays any attention to it. Such disagreements must seem incredulous.

Keep in mind that such arguments about new ideas among doctors are numerous. New theories have a way of stimulating autocratic oppressive behavior that unfortunately stifles the advancement of medicine.

Percy R. Howe, M.D. published a paper stating that he had injected streptococcus bacteria into rabbits and found no adverse reactions in them, thereby directly contradicting Price's work. This article is still being used as proof that root filled teeth can't be of harm to humans. However, the streptococcus bacteria Dr. Howe used in his experiment were the common ones found in the mouth. They usually aren't harmful to us unless they become part of the caries process or of some other disease.

As you learned earlier, upon entering into the dentin tubules and being subjected to medications and root canal fillings, these bacteria radically change and become different organisms. Those that are aerobic lose their usual placid characteristics. They become smaller and anaerobic — that is, they can now live without their usual need for oxygen from air. They also become more virulent, and their toxins more toxic.

Because these organisms, when locked in teeth, did not act in the same manner as the bacteria that cause such infectious diseases as measles, scarlet fever, mumps, pneumonia, etc., it was difficult for some professionals to accept their strange abilities and the very existence of the focal infection process.

Most bacteria need very specific environments in which to thrive — similar to the beaver whose life depends on soft wood trees and the presence of water, or the wildcat family which needs mice and gophers to catch for sustenance. The usual infectious bacteria, despite their devastating ability, have very narrow ranges that govern their existence and the disease entities they cause.

The problem is that we expect focal infection organisms to have similar fixed requirements that govern what they can and cannot do. Probably Dr. Price's greatest contribution was the discovery that focal infection bacteria do not have the usual behavior characteristics of most other organisms.

For the most part, oral bacteria proved to be streptococcal and diplococcal forms. A few other types were found in the mouth but over 90 percent proved to be varieties of the streptococcus family. Furthermore, he learned that their growth and development proceeded according to the media upon which they were growing, but didn't depend on any one kind of sustenance.

The remarkable ability of focal infection bacteria to be polymorphic, that is, to mutate and adapt their lives to the most extreme and unexpected conditions, certainly appears incredible and admittedly quite hard to believe. Who would ever imagine that these tiny microscopic entities would be able to survive, let alone grow luxuriantly, in dentin tubules, in concentrated poisons in boiling water, or autoclaves — all of which stopped and controlled earlier generations of the same species?

These invading warrior organisms, while smaller than the species from which they originated, in proving to be more virile and their toxins more toxic demonstrated their unique ability to drastically adapt to changes in their environment. These attributes allowed them not only to injure their human host but to even cause his or her death.

To a great extent, these invading bacteria are dependent on defects that occur to their host organism. When their host's tissues become traumatically injured, poorly nourished, or partially poisoned, the attack of the organisms occurs more easily and is more potent and deadly. In their effort to conquer, some of these invading organisms generate poisons that paralyze or kill tissues they contact, thereby paving the way for their eventual takeover of that organ or tissue.

Others can live in body tissues without causing any apparent local irritations while they wait for a new home site in some other organ or tissue. Still others of the invading organism species are able to generate toxins either outside or inside cell walls. Some even limit their activity to the cells of the bloodstream.

These numerous attributes of organisms that arise from focal infection sites, whether they be from teeth, tonsils, tonsil tags, sinuses, or any other focal infection source, do cause an infinite variety of local and systemic reactions and conditions.

The concern of my profession is with the effects of dental focal infections. Dr. Price found the organs or tissues that usually become the victim of attack were ones involved with an injury, nutritional deficiency, old age debilitation, or inherited weakness. The lesions that these bacteria usually produced were generally located in what he called the "rheumatic group of organs," causing what he later called the "degenerative diseases."

The organs and tissues most often found to be involved were the heart, eyes, rheumatic and arthritic tissues, kidneys, digestive tract, and nervous system — but he also found that any tissue could be involved. It is the weak link in the body chain that becomes the victim of the attack. The fundamental point of break is the failure of the host's defense mechanisms to ward off attack, that is, the lessening of the efficiency of the immune system.

Getting back to Dr. Percy Howe's rabbits failing to react to his injections of streptococcus bacteria, it should now be easier to see that he was dealing with the bacteria we all have in our mouths on a daily basis. On the other hand, the bacteria Dr. Price's rabbits received were those that were involved inside of infected teeth where they had gone through polymorphic mutation changes and had become more virile and their toxins more toxic.

In spite of the fact that the bacteria Dr. Howe used were not in their virulent form, his criticism of the focal infection theory developed sufficient following to force the information about Dr. Price's research and that of his illustrious colleagues underground.

Another outspoken nonbeliever of Price's work who played a key role in shutting it down was John P. Buckley, Ph.D., D.D.S. He was a personal friend of Dr. Price who admired his honesty and conviction and did credit him with stimulating the spirit of research in dentistry more than any person in our profession.

However, Dr. Buckley believed that because the normal tissues of the body are not always germ free and that with reasonable use of antiseptics and disinfectants dentists seemed to be successful in doing root canal therapy, nothing more was required for success in saving teeth.

Dr. Buckley admitted Dr. Price was making progress in his research efforts but felt he was moving too fast and carried out too many projects. Though he recognized Dr. Rosenow as a bacteriologist of note, he assumed Rosenow knew nothing of dental histopathology.

On the one hand, he states that Drs. Price, Rosenow, Billings, Brophy, Haden, and others were conducting important research. Then too, Dr. Buckley stated: "I do not doubt the bacteriologic findings of men like Price, Rosenow, Haden, and others are correct as far as we understand bacteriology today; but you know and I know that there is something wrong with their conclusions based upon these findings when they talk about the safety of pulpless teeth." That feeling still prevails among most dentists today.

Because a fair number of patients who have root filled teeth removed do not experience health improvements, Dr. Buckley failed to see the significance of the very large numbers who do improve. Dr. Price realized that many factors contributed to the outcome of extractions, including the patient's calcium-phosphorus and acid-base balances. In addition, nutritional and metabolic deficiencies were factors he recognized. Also, different causes could create the same diseases, which complicated the whole issue.

To me it is incredulous that Dr. Buckley could insist that because so many root filled teeth did not show signs of infection or cause degenerative diseases that root filled teeth could not cause systemic infection. Dentists have to wonder how Dr. Buckley could have overlooked the well-known and accepted possibility of infection trapped in lateral accessory canals after a root filling has been placed. The majority of teachers of endodontia teach their students to warn patients of this possibility and to advise them to have follow-up x-ray pictures every year of their root filled teeth to check on the success of the operation.

Not only that, when Dr. Price countered Dr. Buckley's assertions with his extensive research data demonstrating how dental infections upset the calcium-phosphorus and acid-base balances, Dr. Buckley accused him of trying to complicate matters by bringing up something about which he (Buckley) personally knew nothing.

Dr. Buckley also completely ignored the fact that Dr. Price related adverse root fill pathology to the patient's history of susceptibility and to the integrity of the patient's particular biological defense system. Dr. Price was very much concerned about the high and ever-increasing rate of occurrences of degenerative diseases and early deaths resulting therefrom. *He was particularly apprehensive because 75 percent of such people had root canal fillings.*

Dr. Buckley also ignored the fact that Dr. Price was able to demonstrate that 25 percent of those who had root canal fillings, family histories that were free of degenerative illness, and excellent immune systems were able to live to an old age.

Dr. Buckley fought against any acceptance of the focal infection theory because he could not personally visualize a relationship between the bacteria found in the teeth and gums, tonsils, or other mouth tissues as a cause of disease to some other part of the body.

The following is a summary of Dr. Price's comments about the Buckley criticisms:

"People are not living nearly to the entire span of life which they have a right to expect.

Death is occurring even in our most civilized communities largely from the degenerative diseases, chief of which is heart disease.

Even the mortality statistics of our various communities will at this time give an indication of the level and thought of dental practice with regard to the management of infected pulpless teeth.

It is practically, if not entirely, a physical impossibility to sterilize infected cementum by treating through the dentin. It is like trying to sterilize infection in the label on the bottle by putting disinfectants in the bottle.

Root fillings do not continue to fill root canals. The amount of space that ultimately develops is approximately the amount of solvent that was used with the root-filling material, assuming that mechanical filling of every area was possible.

Individuals are not comparable in their defense against degenerative diseases. Some are susceptible and must have an entirely different preventive program.

The degenerative diseases are largely symptoms of degenerative processes in the bloodstream, an important contributing cause for which is long-continued, usually unsuspected, chronic infection.

The roentgen rays (x-rays) cannot reveal all the required information, and under old standards will often be misleading.

The complement fixation method for dental infections can be related to systemic sensitization.

Chronic dental infections reduce the normal bactericidins of the blood.

Leukocytic activity is depressed by chronic dental infections.

Chronic dental infections can produce antigens, to which the sensitized patient may respond with an allergy of severe and very obscure type.

Dental infections can be demonstrated to have had specific localizing ability for many of the organs and tissues of the body. I have already reported on most of these in my papers and books.

> *We cannot, therefore, continue in the light of these new truths to give any quarter to the infected pulpless tooth until we can both accomplish its disinfection and insure its continued sterility."*

In spite of the failure of Dr. Buckley to address the focal infection theory with sound arguments, his words along with those of Dr. Howe's were effective in killing both the acceptance of the Price message about the focal infection diseases and the sale of his books.

Today there has grown to be a general, tacit acceptance of the focal infection theory. Physicians and the American Heart Association strongly urge certain heart disease patients to take antibiotics before and after having any dental treatment — including tooth cleaning — because oral bacteria can so easily be introduced into the bloodstream during dental appointments and cause dreaded endocarditis. Orthopedists who insist that patients with hip or knee replacements take antibiotics before and after dental treatment have found that patients can experience infections in these areas from bacteria traveling from the oral cavity.

It would appear from this that there is now definite belief and concern about the ability of bacteria to establish new infection sites in the body — in other words, acceptance of the focal infection theory. However, there is a false assumption by physicians, dentists, and patients that antibiotics alone can readily control problems of the heart, hips, and knees that so often threaten patients' lives. Sometimes they can, sometimes they can't.

Faith in antibiotics as a cure has allowed physicians, dentists, and the public to forget the basic problems inherent in the presence of a focal infection source. That is, no effort is being made to check patients who are vulnerable for the presence of possible dental infections, such as those from root canal filled teeth and gum infections, as well as those from tonsils, tonsil tags, sinuses, etc.

Not only should these foci sources be repeatedly considered by heart disease patients and their doctors, but also by the average person, for the oral cavity environment is a daily possible source of bacteria which can threaten body organs or tissues.

Most individuals are known to have some degree of gingivitis (gum inflammation) in their mouths. It is not difficult today to picture how the bleeding from the extraction of an infected tooth or other oral procedures can be a way for bacteria to invade the bloodstream and thereby attack an already weakened heart. However it is understandably difficult for heart patients to hear from their doctor that they need antibiotics not only for surgical dental procedures but also for routine prophylaxis.

While bacteremias from dental procedures are usually of short duration and are insignificant to the average person, those people who have had

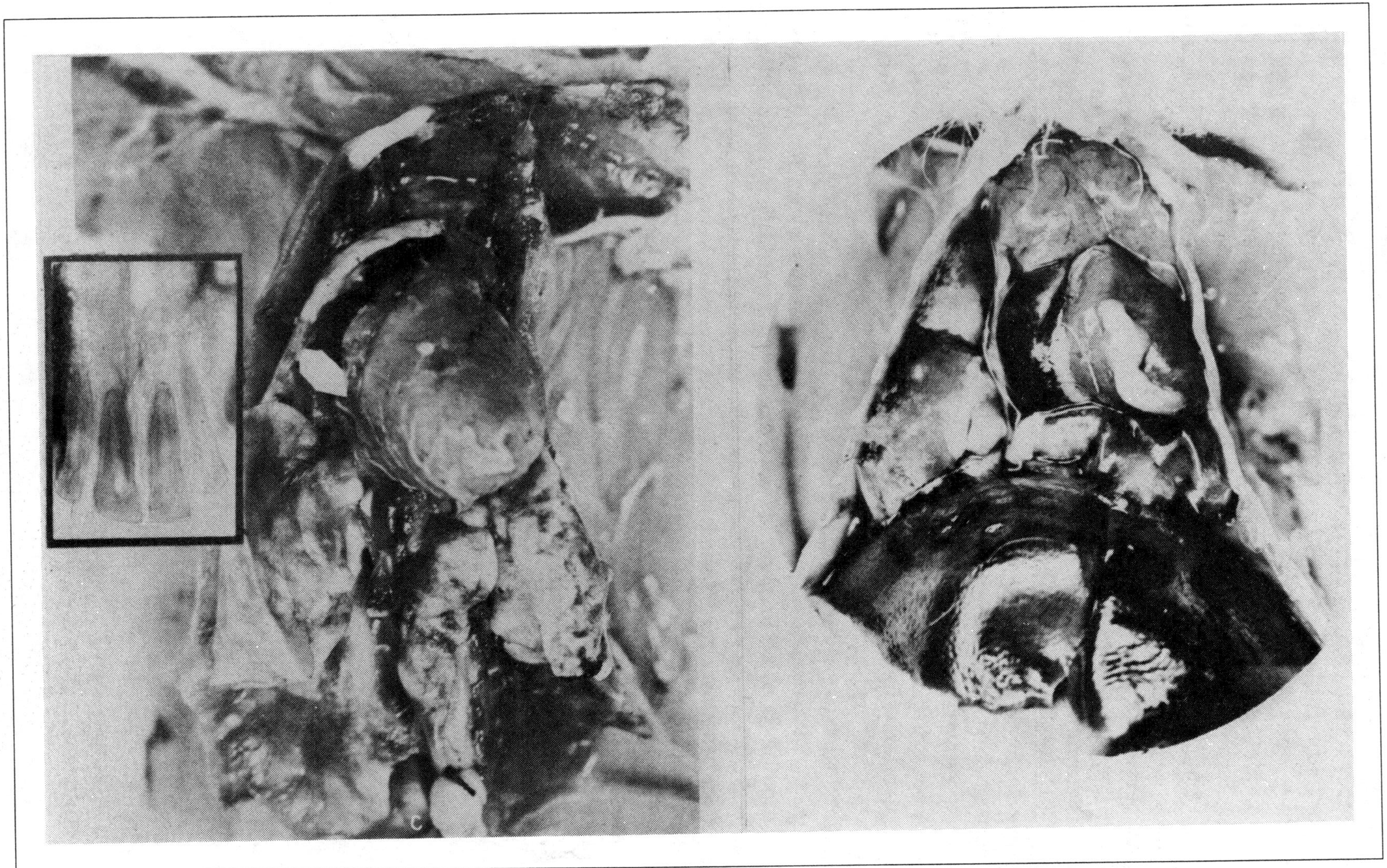

Two rabbits that developed endocarditis from the culture of an apparently healthy central incisor (see insert). This patient was prostrated with the return of a previous acute endocarditis. Price stated that a bacterial focal infection source from streptoccal bacteria could cause a recurrence or worsening of the condition. In this case, one of the apparently healthy central incisors, through the use of thermal and electrical pulp testing, was found to be infected. After the removal of the tooth and a few weeks time, the patient returned to normal activity.

rheumatic fever, rheumatic heart disease, valvular heart disease, etc., must realize that bacteremias, however transient, are potentially very dangerous. This is exactly what Dr. Price demonstrated with his research so long ago.

One of the most severe complications of heart disease is subacute bacterial endocarditis. Before the advent of penicillin, this was almost always fatal. On the preceding page is the picture of a Price rabbit that developed endocarditis from a root filled tooth of a heart patient.

Twenty percent of cases experiencing heart complications after routine dental treatment do so within several weeks after the dental procedures. Because this time lapse is often present, patients usually fail to connect the worsening of their heart condition to their past dental treatment. This is a key reason why such patients must not neglect routine prophylaxis care.

The gum crevices surrounding every tooth, and particularly between teeth, are loaded with bacteria, plus food debris and calculus deposits that also contain bacteria. Some bleeding during scaling and curetting procedures can easily introduce these bacteria and toxins into the bloodstream and result in bacteremia that can seriously damage the heart.

This means that even during tooth brushing, flossing, toothpick use, or chewing hard crusty items of food, it is easy to start minor bleeding that can allow mouth bacteria to be introduced into the bloodstream. Scientific tests have established that bleeding of the gums can cause a high incidence of bacteremia, that is, bacteria in the blood.

The relationship between the transfer of dental bacteria to the heart and the resulting development of infective endocarditis has been directly demonstrated to take place in rabbits by Dr. D.A. McGowan and J.M. Hardie as reported in 1974 in the *British Dental Journal,* and also by Dr. S.L. Bahn in the *Journal of Dental Research*. These two studies confirm Dr. Price's many reports of heart lesions and the transfer of streptococcus bacteria from humans to rabbits.

Inasmuch as there are no antibiotics or combinations of antibiotics that can affect the hundreds of possible different microorganisms found in the mouth that can easily gain entrance into the bloodstream, it behooves physicians and dentists to instruct patients who have heart trouble or body part replacements of their increased vulnerability to all focal infection sources. These patients should be instructed as to the importance of maintaining a high level of oral hygiene care, continued periodontal gum and other dental treatment, and daily meticulous home-care procedures.

Little or no consideration is being given to destroying the majority of mouth bacteria at their source: in the gum crevice. This can be accomplished with local, in the mouth degerming with special mouthwashes and/or topically applied gum disinfectants. These approaches have proven to be more effective than penicillin injections to reduce bacteremias. At least eight major scientific research investigations reporting these findings have been published in such journals as those of the American Dental Association, *Oral Surgery*, *Journal of Dental Research*, *Journal of Endodontics*, etc.

The most successful degerming medicaments and germicidal rinses — those that prevented bactermias to the highest degree — were summarized and reported by I.B. Bender, D.D.S. and Steve Montgomery, D.D.S. in the *Journal of Endodontics*. The very best results of numerous research studies were obtained with topical application into the gum crevice of an iodine-glycerine medicament. No bacteria whatever were found in the blood when it was applied and left to set and act for five minutes before proceeding with planned dental treatment.

Good results were also achieved using 0.5 percent chlorhexadine with 10 percent povidone-iodine solution. If your dentist is not familiar with this study that involves 51 references, he or she can obtain a copy of the article from the American Dental Association Library service.

The acceptance and understanding of how easy it is for bacteremias to occur is, in fact, understanding the focal infection theory in action. This should help everyone to better visualize how bacteria present in the dentin tubules of infected teeth can eventually create such severe illnesses.

In view of the current concern regarding the production of endocarditis and/or knee-hip infections from oral dental sources, a more complete consideration must be given by the medical/dental profession and the public to other ways that focal infections can be induced. A variety of research projects designed to give humans a better chance in their war against focal infection microorganisms must be undertaken.

Summary:

- Suppression of the Dr. Weston Price accomplishments was unfortunate for the development of medicine and detrimental to the health of our people.

- Mainly responsible was a dispute that took place among health professionals as to the validity of the focal infection theory.

- Simply stated, the focal infection theory takes the position that infected teeth, tonsils, tonsil tags, sinuses, and such areas of infection contain bacteria that can travel to another gland, organ or tissue and set up a new infection site.

- Dr. Weston Price was not the only doctor carrying out research on this subject.

- Among the 60 members of the American Dental Association's Research Institute governing body were such famous doctors as Charles Mayo, organizer of the Mayo Clinic; Milton Rosenau, professor of preventive medicine at Johns Hopkins; WilliamWelch, professor of pathology; Frank Billings who gave focal infection its name; Truman Brophy, dental school dean; Frank Lillie, professor of zoology and embryology; and Victor Vaughan, medical department dean and American Medical Association president.

- As in so many disputes about medical discoveries, even though the majority of leading doctors believed in the focal infection theory, these leading scientists were overidden and silenced.

- The fight *against* the focal infection theory was mainly carried out by doctors Percy Howe and John Buckley.
  * Howe based his opposition on a study he conducted injecting rabbits with the normal placid streptococcus bacteria secured from the mouth, not bacteria from an infection site or a root filled tooth.
  * In his investigation, none of the animals became sick or died.
  * Buckley was unable to see how infected teeth that showed excellent evidence of bone repair after root canal therapy could possibly still be infected. Then too, because some who had root filled teeth removed did not recover, he questioned the validity of the conclusion that a percentage of patients did get well due to the removal of a tooth or teeth.

- The arguments of these two men were weak and they failed to consider or believe
  * That poor nutrition and inherited genetic problems are also causes of degenerative diseases.
  * That oral bacteria do not act in the same manner as do the germs that cause measles, smallpox, mumps, scarlet fever, etc.
  * That when teeth become infected, oral bacteria find the dentin tubules an ideal cave-like hiding place, and that these germs and their toxins — like the viruses that cause cancer — metastasize and escape to infect hearts, joints, kidneys, lungs, the stomach, eyes, and countless other tissues.
  * That what makes these bacteria so dangerous is their ability to become polymorphic, that is to mutate, adapt, change, become smaller, anaerobic, more virulent and more toxic.
  * That pregnant women or others experiencing a higher than normal degree of stress become particularly susceptible to diseases arising from oral infection sources.

- By the mid-thirties, most physicians and dentists believed the focal infection theory to be correct and valid.

- With the advent of penicillin, there arose the belief that antibiotics could cure all these problems and little is heard today about focal infections.
- However, the fact is that antibiotics can't get inside the dentin tubules once a tooth loses its blood supply due to root canal treatment. If antibiotics can't get inside tubules, they can't kill the bacteria therein.
- The focal infection theory, while rarely talked about today, is paid great heed to by physicians and dentists of heart patients and those with hip and knee replacements. Because of the ease of bacteremias occurring during dental treatment, including routine teeth cleaning, these patients are given prescriptions for antibiotics.
- Even the smallest amount of bleeding in the mouth will cause oral bacteria to get into the bloodstream.
- Degerming methods presented by dentists Bender and Montgomery in the *Journal of Endodontics* prevent bacteremias to a higher degree than have antibiotics.
- In the interest of all heart and hip or knee replacement patients, these degerming procedures deserve greater attention than they are currently receiving.
- Such patients should be carefully assessed for the presence of infected teeth, germs, tonsils, or other focal infection sources if endocarditis and other infections are to be prevented.

CHAPTER 18

The Degenerative Diseases Caused by Tooth Infections
Case Histories

Quite often Price referred to the high number of "rheumatic group lesions" that resulted from dental infections. That terminology produced some confusion as it placed extreme emphasis on rheumatism and arthritis. Although rheumatic and arthritic illnesses often result from oral infections, they aren't any more prevalent as a result of dental infections than those that affect the heart and circulatory system.

Toward the end of Volume I of his *Dental Infections, Oral and Systemic,* Price made this statement:

> *"It seems probable that we will come more and more to speak of them as the degenerative diseases, since they constitute the slow loss of function, with structural degeneration, of various organs and tissues of the body. The government statistics speak of them frequently as old age diseases, and it is pathetic that so many individuals are slowly dying of old age anywhere from thirty years on."*

Time has proven him correct, as the term degenerative disease is now fairly well understood and is frequently used by the public. For the most part, throughout the book I have dropped Dr. Price's references to the term "rheumatic group."

At the time of Dr. Price's research, most people thought that degenerative diseases resulted from accidental exposure of the body to specifically different organisms, each of which attacked either the heart, the kidneys, the joints, etc. — much like catching measles or mumps. Today that feeling is still a predominant one, but it is accompanied by the realization that many organ and tissue diseases can be due to nutritional and/or metabolic disorders and breakdowns as well.

The most powerful force driving me to report Dr. Price's work to America and the world is the fact that many people are suffering severe ill health, and even premature death, because of these dental and other focal infections. By Dr. Price's simple experiment of placing root filled or other infected teeth under the skin of rabbits, he has given us an iron clad method to demonstrate whether a tooth sterilization method is successful.

I trust that not only lay readers but the medical and dental professions as well will, at long last, recognize how easily focal infections in teeth, tonsils or other tissues can be transferred to other organs and tissues and can end up causing endocarditis in hearts, nephritis in kidneys, and a whole host of other devastating illnesses. While not all root canal treatments result in the transference of disease, keep in mind that over 24 million root canal operations were performed last year and most of these surgeries could have been prevented had the initial cavity in the tooth been discovered earlier.

In view of the ever-growing cost of health care that is bankrupting many families and is similarly threatening our government, very serious reappraisals of Dr. Price's research by the dental profession is called for in an effort to eliminate the huge number of degenerative diseases that are related to focal infection sources.

What you know now, and what should be public knowledge, is that *there is a much higher incidence of the occurrence of degenerative disease in those who have root canal fillings and periodontal gum disease than in those who maintain a healthy mouth*. We must accept the fact that bacteria find our tissues so attractive and desirable that they mutate and change form in order to survive there. At the same time we cannot ignore nutritional and metabolic effects upon our immune systems.

Dr. Price reported that, in a large number of cases, even when root filled teeth that appeared perfectly normal and without symptoms were extracted, a high percentage of the patients who had been experiencing heart problems found their conditions totally or almost totally subsided.

The physicians who understand the harmful role teeth can play in their patient's lives will, I trust, keep in mind that none of this information in any way condones the wholesale condemnation of all teeth. Early in my practice I was horrified to find a number of patients whose physicians took the focal infection theory too literally and advised them to have all their teeth out, teeth that were in no way involved in their arthritic condition.

Because dentists construct dentures that look and act so much like natural teeth, people have come to believe that they are just as good as their own. While dentures are among the best of all body replacement parts, they are in no way as good at masticating food as natural teeth in good repair. Most patients with full dentures are enthused about them and insist that they can eat everything.

Having checked diet intakes, however, I have found that when a denture patient can't chew certain foods, those foods are gradually dropped from their diet and replaced with foods they can chew. In time, the diets of many are composed of only soft foods that require little mastication ability. Most of the soft varieties chosen are of poor nutritional quality.

Some patients even plead with dentists to take out healthy teeth, based on a belief that they will then be through with the need for the expense of dental care. The fact is that most people's poor nutritional habits cause their gums to keep shrinking away, necessitating the relining of their dentures. This can only be done once or twice before new dentures are required. Each new set of teeth means that the gum ridge foundation that supports the load of chewing is continuing to shrink. The answer to all this is to save natural teeth; that is, to "prevent decay the proven way" by eliminating junk foods and replacing them with natural ones.

Getting back to degenerative diseases, there are so many that I won't try to list them all here. The most common ones that Dr. Price found could be transferred from patient to rabbits from infected teeth involved arthritis; rheumatism; heart lesions; kidney, liver and gall bladder problems; neck, back and shoulder stiffness; eyes; ears; skin; shingles; anemia; pneumonia; appendicitis; neuritis, neuralgia, and nervous system breakdowns; and hardening of the arteries.

Further discussion of how degenerative diseases were found to be involved follow. Endocarditis and myocarditis heart problems, along with circulatory system involvements, were discussed in Chapter 12. Some others are:

EYE INFECTIONS

Eye infections transferred to rabbits from patients with eye diseases was very dramatic. The accompanying picture "C" shows a woman patient's eye condition. She had a history of five such attacks with progressive severity over a two year period. Picture "D" shows teeth which appeared normal on x-ray film. "A" shows the rabbit two days after inoculation of a culture of bacteria from the tooth. Figure "B" is the rabbit's eye after 72 hours. Only one of the rabbit's eyes was involved. After the offending teeth were involved.

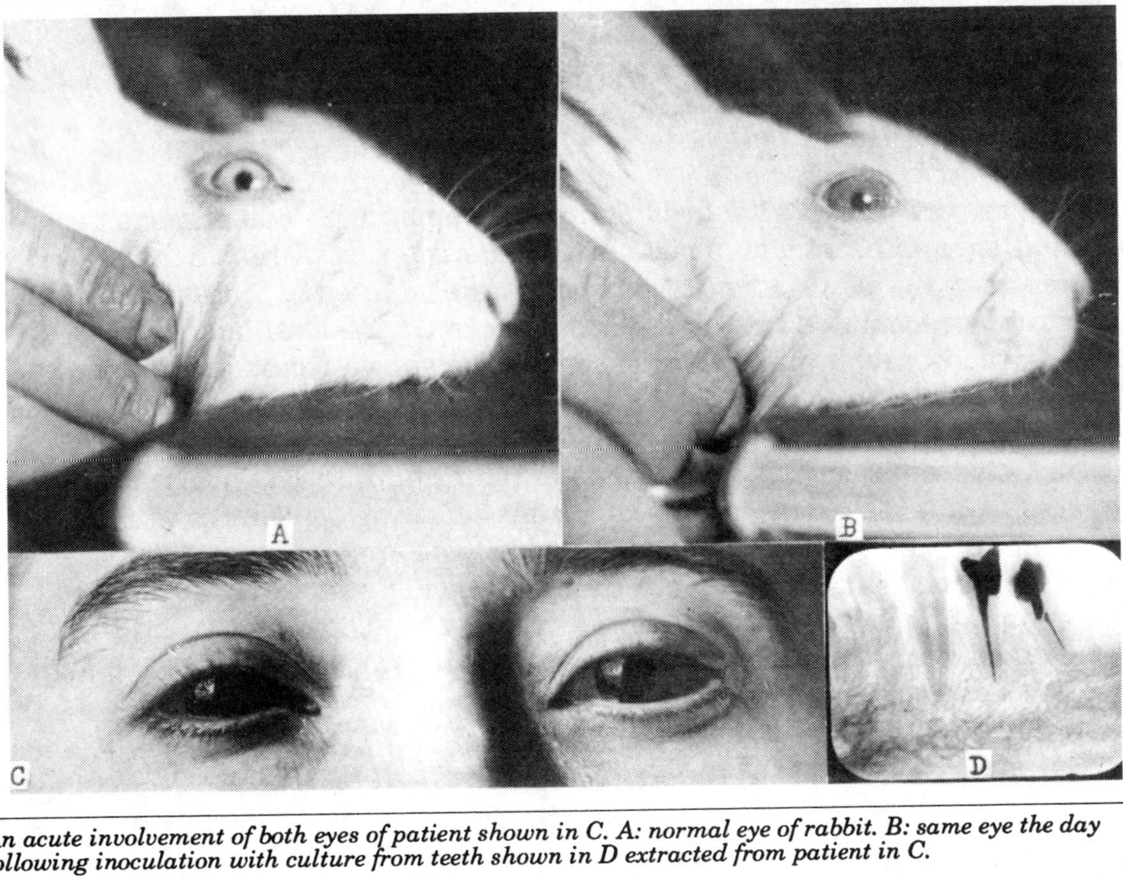

An acute involvement of both eyes of patient shown in C. A: normal eye of rabbit. B: same eye the day following inoculation with culture from teeth shown in D extracted from patient in C.

After the offending teeth were extracted from the patient, the acute inflammation she suffered was markedly reduced and was nearly gone in three days. She had no recurrence of the trouble after three years.

Dr. Price found that a variety of eye problems of patients were readily transferred to rabbits and many became severe enough in the rabbits to cause the loss of sight.

KIDNEY TROUBLE

Originally Dr. Price believed kidney infections to be only remotely related to dental focal infections. He eventually found, however, that many 30 to 40 year olds were developing nephritis (kidney disease) without the disease being suspected by the patient or the physician. Invariably, these patients were also found to have definite dental infections. Below is an x-ray picture of a tooth under a rabbit's skin from a patient with kidney trouble.

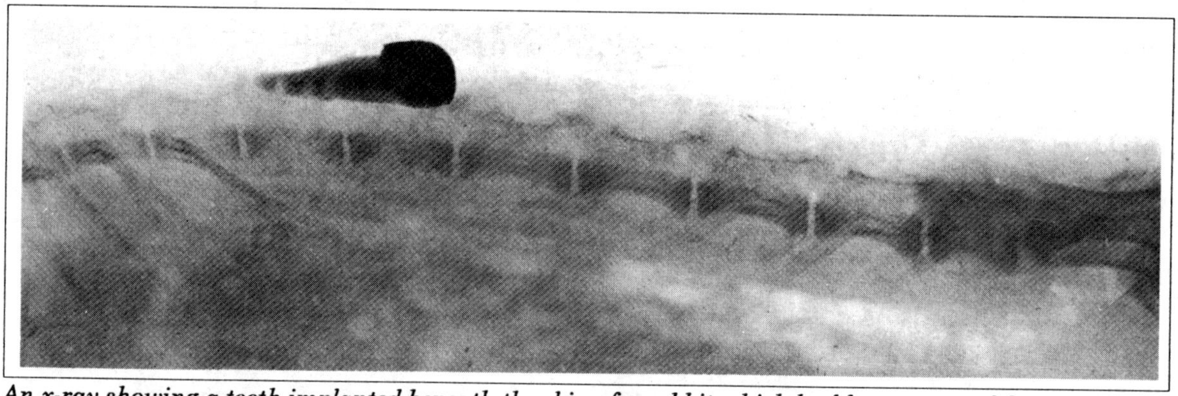

An x-ray showing a tooth implanted beneath the skin of a rabbit which had been removed from a patient suffering from nephritis.

The case report of a 41 year old married woman who was suffering from rheumatism and heart trouble is of particular interest. A routine urine analysis also disclosed kidney involvement. Her extracted tooth was cultured and a rabbit inoculated in a vein with one cc of the 24-hour old culture. After 49 days, the ill rabbit died; autopsy results are shown in the pictures on the opposite page.

These pictures show that the rabbit's two kidneys were enlarged enormously (compare with normal one to the right of the large right kidney). Pictures "A" and "B" show microscopic views of dying cells and a great number of dilated tubules of glomeruli (clusters of cells) that appear like a cystic condition. The patient's lassitude, rheumatism, and nephritis all cleared up promptly on removal of her two lower infected teeth, and there was no recurrence of former severe symptoms for three years, even though the patient was carrying a heavy work overload.

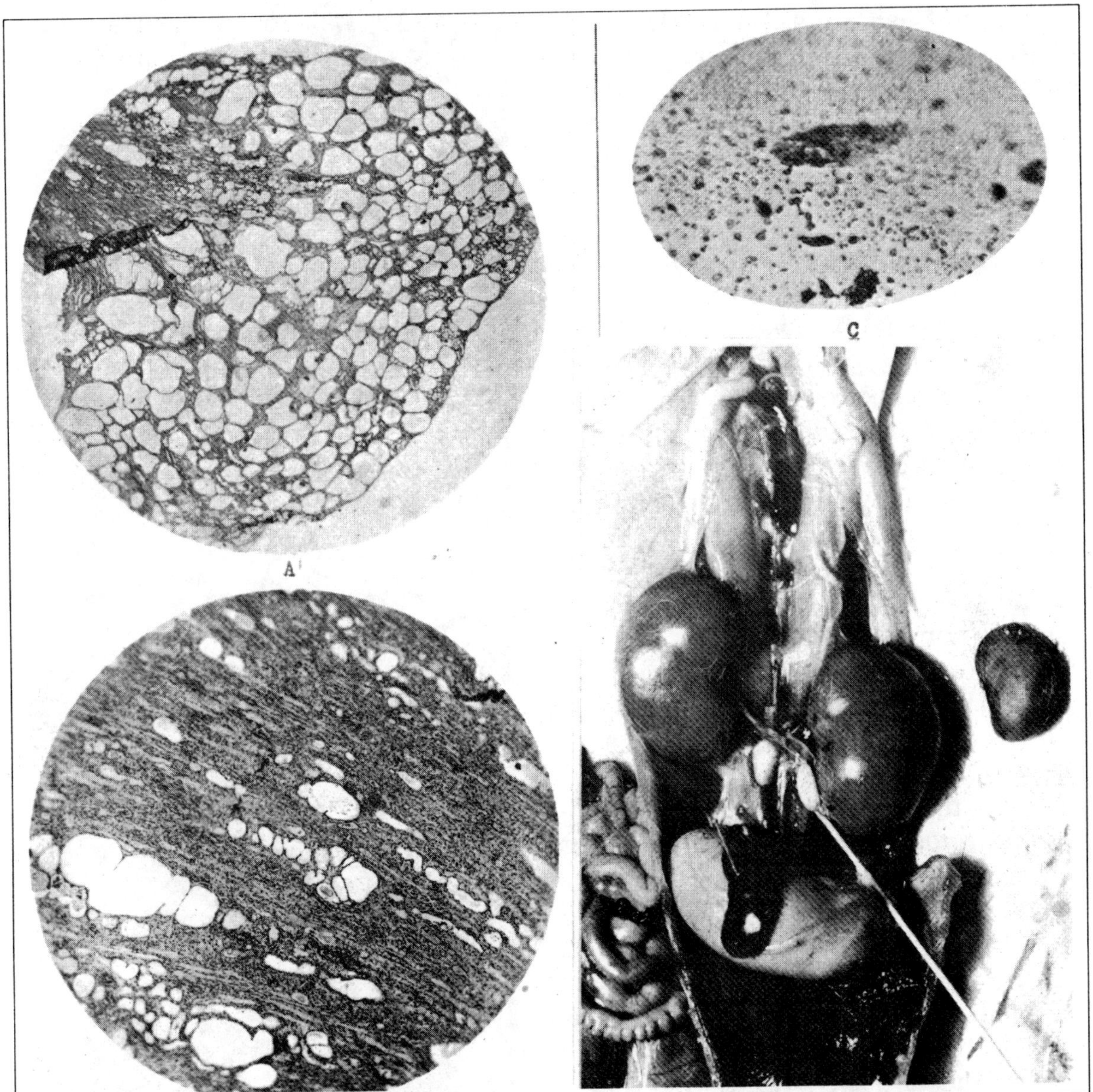

Acute interstitial nephritis produced in a rabbit. A and B: tissue sections showing cellular necrosis and edema. D: both kidneys of injected rabbit five times normal size. See normal kidney to right, also hypertrophy of adrenals. C: casts from patient's urine.

STOMACH ULCERS

Case Number 965 concerned a 43 year old woman who had virtually been an invalid for six years suffering from nervousness, neuritis, and nervous indigestion. These symptoms were associated with neuralgic pains that

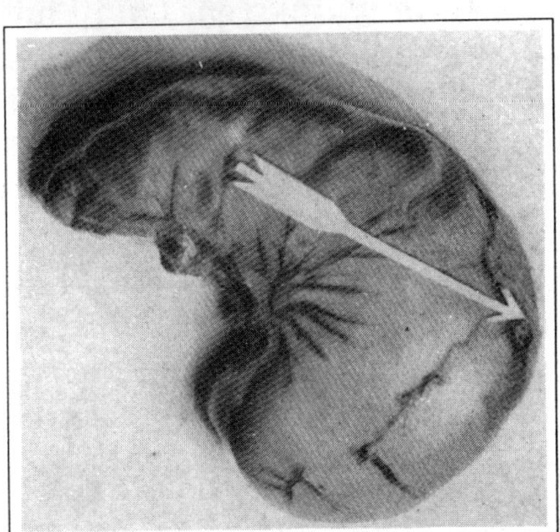

Stomach ulcer perforation.

occurred at her waistline. Such cases were usually grouped together as alimentary tract and associate organ lesions, as they involved the digestive tract, the gall bladder, stomach, intestinal indigestion, and the appendix.

Because this patient had a most severe amount of condensing osteitis (dense bone just below the roots), and such cases usually showed little x-ray evidence of infection, all of her upper teeth were removed. This brought a prompt improvement in the patient's health that allowed her to return to previous activities.

Most dentists would say that even though this patient had severe osteitis, her root canal fillings appeared satisfactory and the root of the upper left second bicuspid appears relatively easy to treat. However, a culture taken from these other teeth and inoculated into a rabbit produced the ulcer you see in the accompanying picture.

Other than the retained upper bicuspid root of this patient, most dentists who do endodontic treatments would have misjudged the extent of the infection present in these teeth and their relationship to the patient's six years of ill health that cleared on removal of her upper teeth.

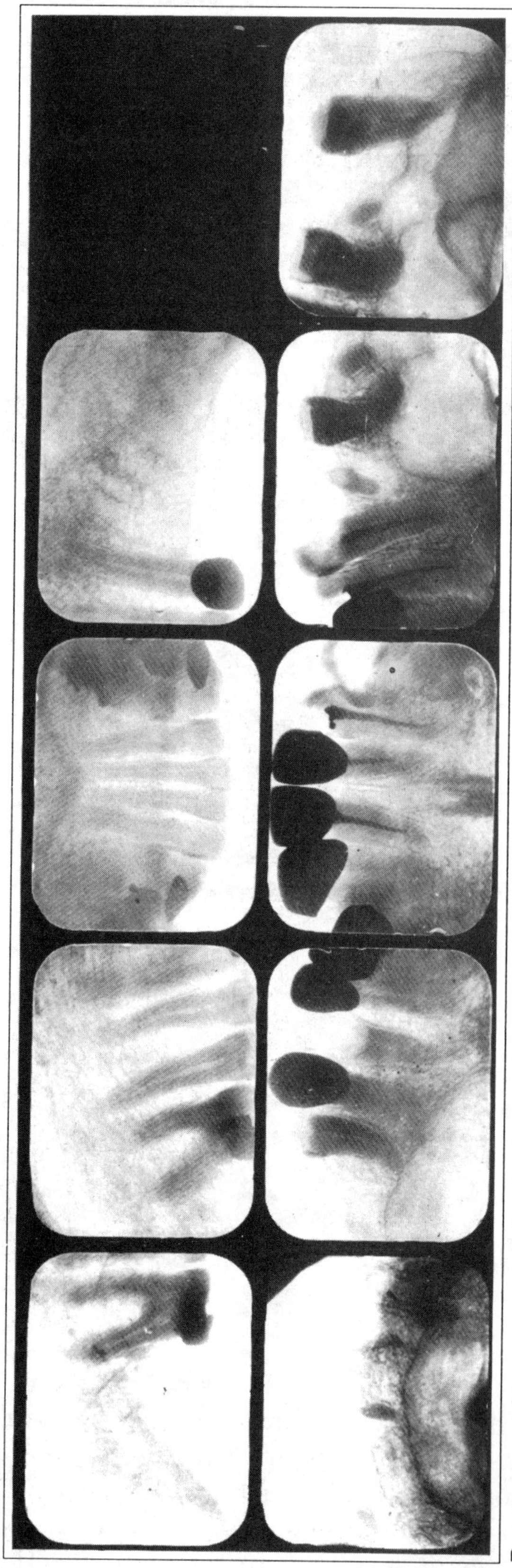

Roentgenographic appearance of teeth of stomach ulcer case.

OVARIAN CYSTS

Quite lacking in medical and dental literature of Dr. Price's time was any teaching about acute and chronic infections of the sex organs, or any mention of their relationship to focal infection. Dr. Price found that a large number of women with ovarian gland difficulties had infected teeth, or teeth that contained root canal fillings.

Even though most women made excellent recoveries when infected teeth were removed, Dr. Price stated that he could not determine whether the bacteria had an ability to select a woman's ovaries, tubes, and uterus or whether their presence aggravated and worsened already compromised tissues. Over a thousand rabbits were used to study the causes of these frequent female problems.

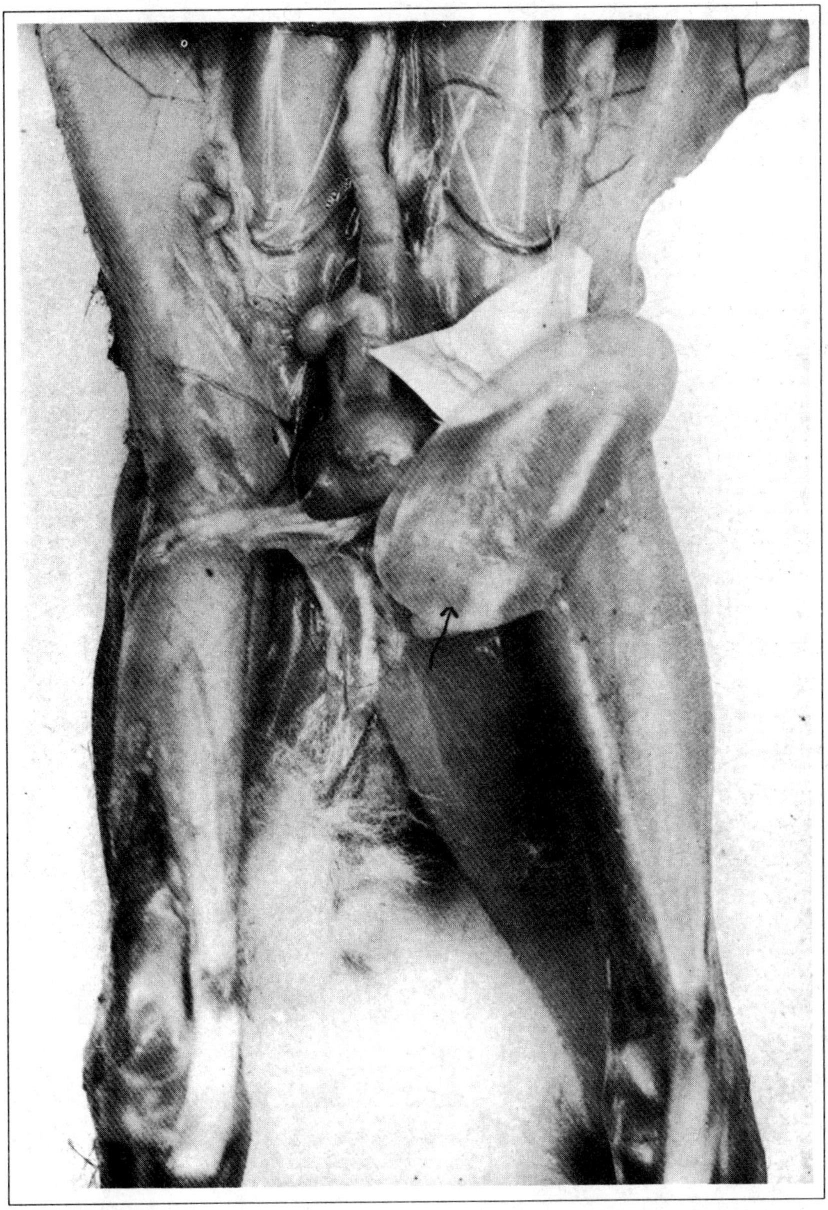

A very large ovarian cyst produced in a rabbit from a dental culture.

The history of Case Number 185 is a good example of the many cases investigated. This concerns a 20 year old unmarried woman whose distress at the time of her menstrual period was so severe that she was bed-ridden for several days. In time it became obvious that her physical and mental health was being seriously hampered.

Review of the history of her difficulties showed that some five years previously she was hit by a golf ball over her left ovary. She did not think the event significant as there was no evidence of local injury and only a short period of discomfort. At the time she did have some infected teeth which she carried during the intervening period.

As her condition deteriorated more and more, it became necessary for this patient to solve her health problems or give up her university work. In addition to the menstrual disturbances, she also suffered an acute nervous condition that affected her breathing and was followed by numbness and a severe pain in the back of the neck which worsened just before the start of her periods.

The patient had a root canal filling on her two front teeth that appeared satisfactory but a lower molar had an obvious large infection. She improved markedly upon the removal of the molar but in a few months her health became compromised again.

After removal of her two front teeth, she gained weight and her mental and physical impairments improved markedly.

Cultures made from these two teeth were inoculated into four female rabbits and two males. All of the females developed acute infections of their ovaries and tubes. The males remained healthy.

This operation made such a great change in her health that her mother stated she was like a new and entirely different person both mentally and physically. Her menstrual periods became normal and free of pain. She gained back lost weight and had no return of trouble in the following two years up to the recording of these events.

TESTICAL INFECTIONS

The picture below is of the acutely inflamed and swollen testicles of three rabbits that had been inoculated with cultures from three different teeth of a patient who had, for several months prior to the extractions, experienced painful swelling of his own testicles that was thought to be related to a rheumatic involvement. Both his rheumatism and testicular pain were greatly relieved by the removal of the infected teeth.

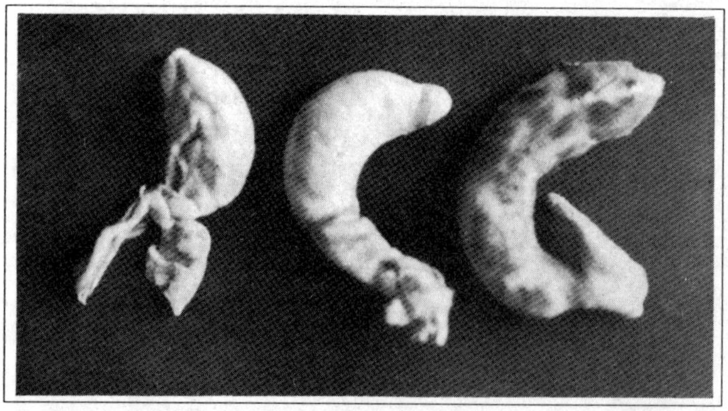

Acutely inflamed testicles, one from each of three rabbits inoculated from the cultures of three different teeth of a patient suffering from acute swelling and pain in testicles. He had previously had gonorrheal or syphilitic infection.

The patient acknowledged that some 20 years prior to that time he had been treated for a gonorrheal or syphilitic infection.

In tests of some hundred rabbits, only a few developed these testicular involvements, although other glands and tissues did become involved.

BLADDER INFECTION

Irritations of the bladder were frequently found to be caused by dental infections. One such case involved a man of 65 who was so distressed with cystitis that for five years he had been unable to leave his home as he had to void urine every 30 to 60 minutes or his distress was unbearable. His sleep was particularly disturbed.

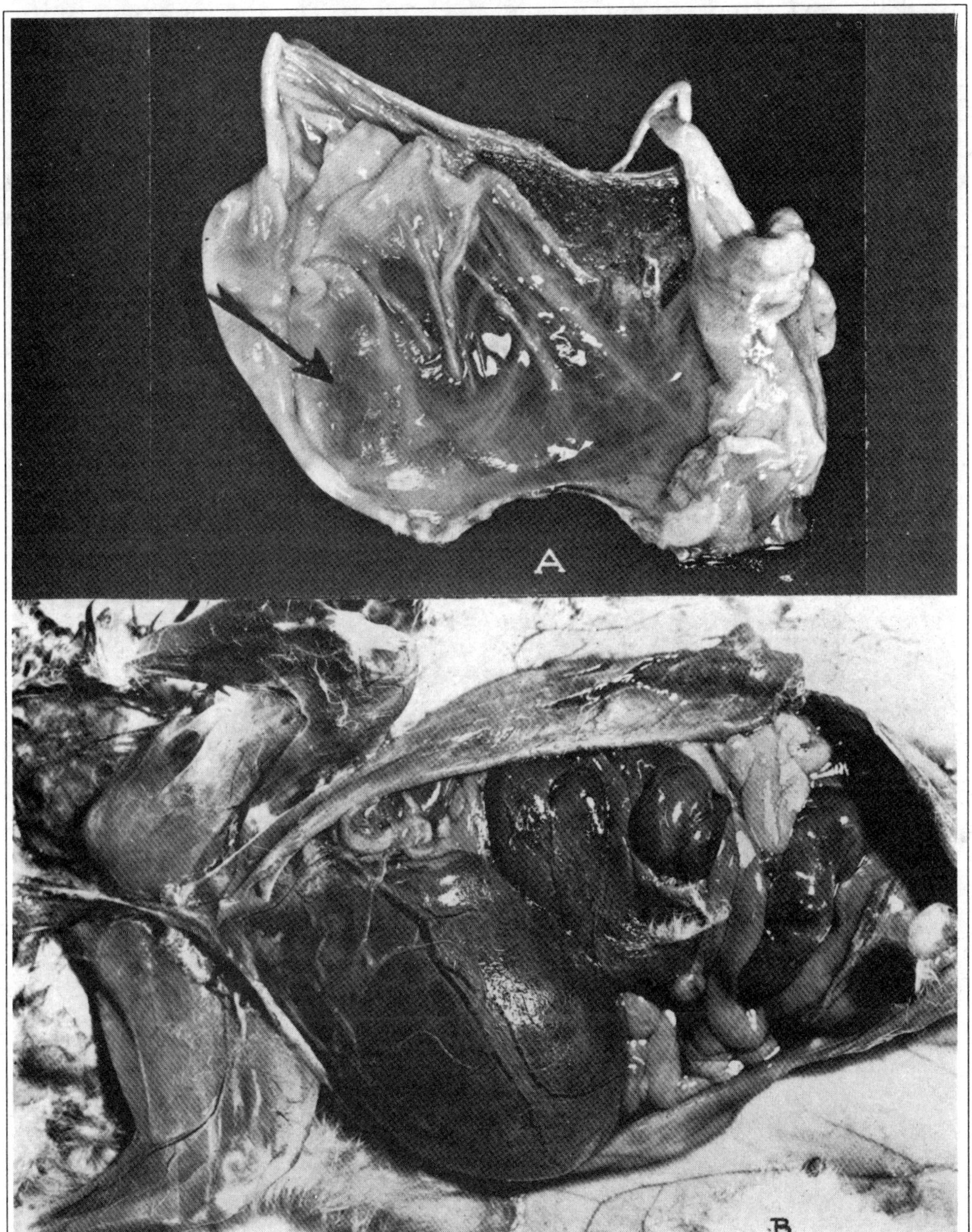

Paralysis of the bladder with urine retention produced in a rabbit by dental infection. A shows deep ulcer on inner surface of distended bladder. Bladder shown in B is 20 times normal size.

This man's staphyloccal bladder infection (preceding page) improved in 24 hours upon removal of two lower infected molar teeth. In two weeks he was able to retain urine for five hours.

CHOREA—HYPERACTIVITY

St. Vitus dance or chorea are old technical terms for what we call hyperactivity or "attention deficit disorder" today. The dictionary definition is: "irregular, spasmodic involuntary movements of the limbs and/or facial muscles."

So that you do not assume this is a condition only of modern times, I will draw your attention to the following case. The patient's history is such an important contribution to parents considering the possibility of the presence of similar focal infection in their children that I am going to quote it just as it appeared in Volume II of Price's *Dental Infections and Degenerative Diseases:*

> *"Case No. 458 – The patient, nine years of age, was brought by his mother with the following history. As the tears streamed down her cheeks, she said, 'Why have my husband and I been cursed with such a wicked boy? The teacher sent him home with a note saying that if he returns she will leave the school.*
>
> *'He cannot play with children without slapping them in the face or some other unpardonable violence without provocation. He does this also to his father and to me. While keeping him out of school, since we have to, I thought it would be a good time to have his teeth taken care of, etc., etc.'*
>
> *We made a few studies of the boy and soon found that he had largely lost his power of coordination. He had a very sharply developed symptom group chorea with an exaggeration of the irritability phase. While undertaking to make roentgenograms of his teeth, he would strike me in the face without any provocation.*
>
> *In addition to making these studies, we made motion pictures of his lack of coordination. It was apparently impossible for him to sit still, and every moment he was twitching and jerking and, as such patients do, would try to turn an involuntary muscular contraction into a voluntary one. He would find his knee jerking up, and, in order to avoid the embarrassment, would turn it into a kick; and similarly with his hands. If he had something in his hand at the time the involuntary reflex occurred, and his hand started swinging, he would let the article fly as though he had intended that to be the movement.*

We do not wonder that his teacher had reached the limit of her capacity to control, for no ordinary power could control him, not even his own mind. We explained to the mother that her boy was not a bad boy; that he had an infection of the cortex of the brain, probably largely coming from his infected teeth; and that when his infection was removed he probably would return to normal.

With very great difficulty, because of his extreme condition, we succeeded in removing the deciduous teeth which were deeply carious, several of which had infected pulps. These were cultured and animals were inoculated, several of which developed very acute involvements of the central nervous system; and we had four at one time of this series with such marked central nervous system disturbance that with little excitement they would fall on their sides.

Sections made from the cortex of the brain of one such rabbit showed multiple petechial pin point bleeding points and diplococcal zone hemorrhages which would lead to irritability and impetuosity, and even violence, all of which so often make up the picture of chorea."

Immediately after the removal of these teeth, the boy's condition improved and he returned to normal very rapidly. In two weeks' time he was back in school, a normal child, and has not had a single recurrence in five years.

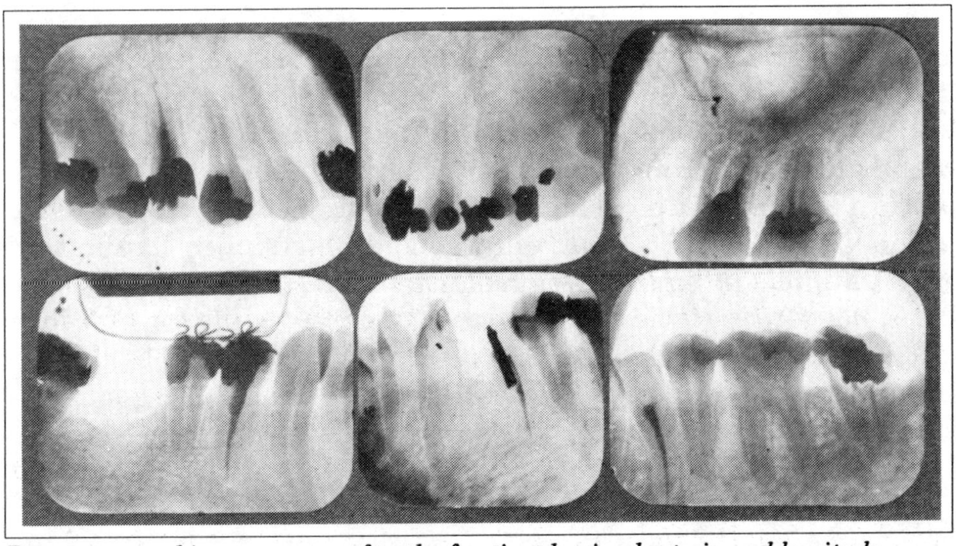

Roentgenographic appearance of teeth of patient having hysteria and lassitude.

Before learning from Price that infected teeth could be a cause of hyperactivity, I had some success treating such children as part of my caries prevention diet analysis program by getting them off of sugar and junk foods and replacing these foods with good diets and nutritional supplements. Nutritional treatment invariably produced miraculous results. Dr. Ben Feingold's fine research into the effect of certain chemical additives in food points to another cause of hyperactivity. It is a sad commentary but many parents of hyperactive children, said to be three to five percent of all children, find the prescription for the drug Ritalin easier to handle than changing the family's dietary habits.

One parent who brought his child to me for nutritional counseling said that treatment with Ritalin was a disaster. Her son became a zombie, couldn't sleep, had bad dreams when he did — but worst of all, he became very violent at times.

There is a general feeling that these children will grow out of their hyperactivity but there are adults, though somewhat in control, who just can't sit still but must be moving about all of the time.

In view of the experience of Dr. Price with such children, it would seem that the first step for a parent would be to find out whether their child has any infected teeth, tonsils, tonsil tags, or other sources of focal infection.

DIGESTIVE TRACT: INTESTINE, COLON, APPENDIX, GALL BLADDER

About the disturbances of the digestive tract, Dr. Price reported that none of the many different kinds of illnesses prove more obscure as to their cause than those of the large and small intestines. Time after time they found the patients' symptom history included very accute diarrhea, constipation and acute colitis.

These cases were found to be related to both root canal infections and those of the gums as well. Such cases were of particular interest as they so often produced similar symptoms in the animals inoculated with germs from the teeth and gums of patients who had these symptoms.

The picture on the next page shows an enfolding of the inflamed intestine into the colon, appendicitis, and an enlarged gall bladder in a rabbit originating from a patient's infected lower molar tooth.

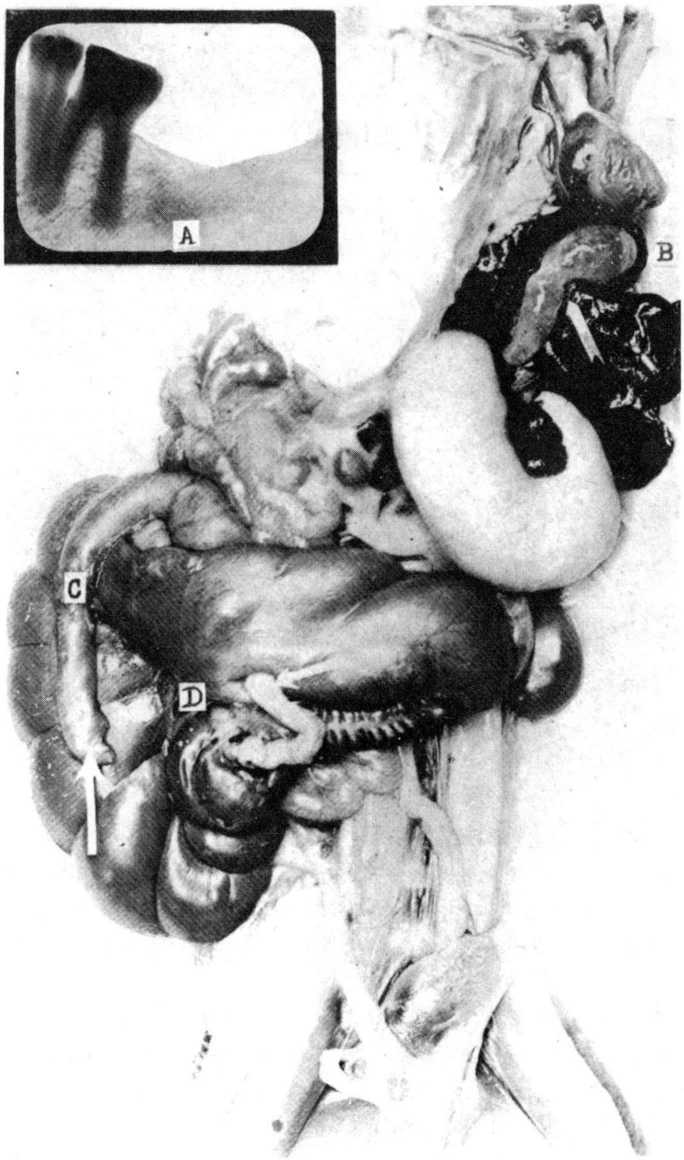

Digestive tract involvements of rabbit
A: non-vital molar;
B: gall bladder involvement;
C: acute appendicitis;
D: an inflammatory invagination of the cecum into the colon.

Many readers will feel that with the use of today's antibiotics' infections in teeth are able to be arrested. There is no question antibiotics have saved many lives through their ability to control bacteria. However, the germs trapped in the dentin tubules of teeth by root canal fillings are another matter.

Inasmuch as the dentin tubules lose their blood supply connection when nerves are removed from teeth, antibiotics are unable to reach the bacteria to eradicate them.

Summary:

- Dr. Price's decision to call all diseases resulting from dental infections "degenerative diseases" was a prophetic one. Time has proven him correct and people generally recognize that this term implies a progressive health deterioration.

- During Dr. Price's time and even today, people believe that degenerative diseases are caused by accidental exposure to specific germs and as a result the heart, kidneys, joints, etc. are attacked — much like contracting the measles, mumps, chicken pox, etc.

- Because, in some cases, bacteria are involved, the above view still predominates. The issue is further confused by the fact that tissue deterioration also takes place due to nutritional deficiencies and excesses.

- At the same time, hardly anyone realizes the extent to which focal infections from teeth, tonsils and tonsil tags are major contributors to the presence of degenerative diseases. That fact motivated the writing of this book.

- It is most difficult on one hand to realize how fabulous the contributions of the dental profession have been in preserving and extending the life of teeth — and on the other hand to recognize that the need for root canal fillings is a distinct indication of failure to discover tooth decay when it starts, rather than when it is so deep that the pulp has become infected.

- Then too, had this very revealing research of Dr. Price's not been buried, there is a good chance that by now we would have solved the problems of how to sterilize the bacteria trapped in dentin tubules.

- It is extremely disturbing to think about all the degenerative diseases that exist and are bankrupting our people and our country. Worst of all is the fact that so many people are dying of afflictions that could be alleviated.

- In this chapter about degenerative diseases, I have included some of the more common ones Dr. Price presented in his two books and pictures of these conditions.

- The degenerative diseases mentioned in this chapter with accompanying pictures were:

* Eye infections: picture of a patient, rabbit, and tooth x-ray
* Kidney disease (nephritis): picture of a kidney swollen to five times its normal size
* Stomach ulcer: picture of ulcer perforation and x-ray pictures of the offending teeth
* Ovarian cysts: one very large one
* Testicles: acute pain and swelling
* Bladder: paralysis, ulceration and swelling to 20 times its normal size
* Chorea: now called hyperactivity or attention deficit disorder (A parent's account of a 9 year old is presented.)
* Hysteria and lassitude: x-ray pictures demonstrate the cause in one patient

- These examples should give you some idea about the thousands of different degenerative disease cases that were extensively studied.

- Because Dr. Price's investigations indicate that those who have root canal fillings and/or periodontal gum disease have a higher incidence of degenerative diseases than those free of such conditions, it behooves us to adopt sound preventive measures in our day-to-day lives.

- Should you have a degenerative disease that is defying your physician's best efforts, you might present him/her with a copy of this book. Only your physician or dentist is in a position to assess what is best for you regarding the removal of root filled or possibly infected teeth.

- If removal of a tooth or teeth is decided upon, please read Chapter 25 carefully as it contains the protocol for romoval of infected tissue that might otherwise remain in the tooth's socket.

CHAPTER 19

The Wonders of Surgery
The Apicoectomy

When a tooth that has had a root canal filling develops a granuloma, cyst or some other infected area at the end of the root, dentists will sometimes endeavor to save the tooth by performing an operation called apicoectomy. The area of infection that is seen on x-ray pictures is actually a hole in the bone of the jaw that has been eaten away by bacteria and toxins. It contains pus, bacteria, and infected tissue.

The apicoectomy surgery is done using a local anesthetic. An incision is made in the gum and the dentist enters into the infected area and curettes away the diseased tissue.

In order to be able to remove all infected tissue surrounding a tooth's root end, it is sometimes necessary to also remove a portion of the tooth's root end (apex). This is done with a surgical dental burr or drill. The term apicoectomy was adopted because the end tip of the root is so often removed during this procedure.

Two or three stitches are used to close the wound. These areas experience some swelling for two or three days but generally heal with very little discomfort. Usually new bone immediately begins to grow and fill in the jaw at the end of the root, and after six to 12 months one can no longer distinguish the location of the infection sight. In other words, the area's appearance is now normal.

At times when cysts or other large areas of infection are found, dentists will elect to do the root canal treatment and apicoectomy at the same sitting. Generally I preferred doing both procedures simultaneously as it was much easier to clean out the root canal that way. In addition, we could spray a disinfectant through the root canal and vacuum the debris and infected material out from the root end surgical area. It was also easier to get a good dense root canal filling as any overpacking could easily be removed.

In my practice I did a fair number of these apicoectomy surgeries and I cannot recall any that did not show full healing at the end of the root of the tooth, usually within the period of one year. We were not universally successful with teeth treated nonsurgically.

A couple of case history reports from my files will allow you to see how well infections responded to the apicoectomy procedure.

The first is of a woman who came home from on a trip to Mexico with severe diarrhea and intestinal involvement. When a leading Beverly Hills gastroenterologist was unable to cure her intestinal infection, the patient, knowing I was doing nutritional counseling, sought my opinion.

Oral examination didn't indicate any obvious pathologic conditions or tooth decay, but there were many fillings present. Full mouth x-ray examination disclosed large abscesses from accessory canals on both of her upper lateral incisors (the teeth next to the two front teeth).

The original x-ray pictures and surgery took place in March of 1955. The last follow-up x-ray was February, 1976: 21 years later. To my knowledge, she still has those teeth.

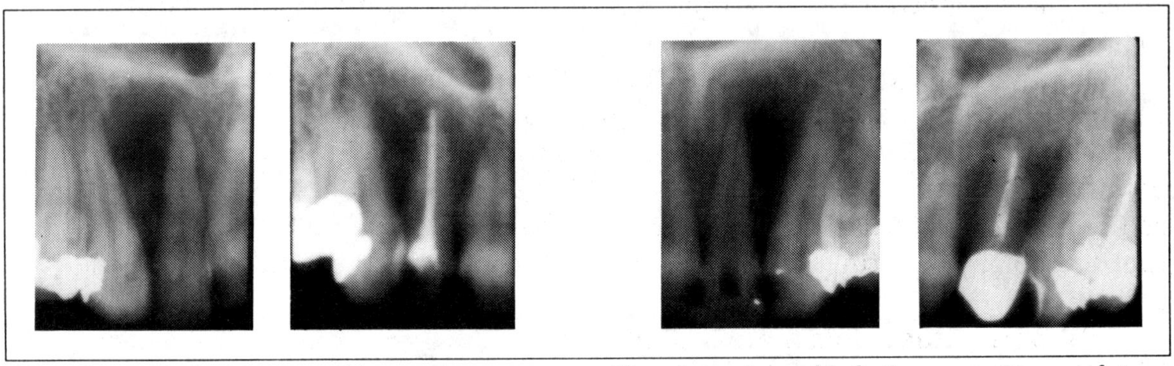

Huge lateral infection. *21 years later.* *Huge lateral canal infection .* *21 years later.*

With hindsight and the information we have gained from Dr. Price's research, one can see that the failure of the physician's treatment in this case was no doubt due to the hidden focal infection arising from these two teeth that had spread to her intestines. The patient's improvement was so dramatic that she claimed I had saved her life.

Though I believe the infected teeth played a supporting role in her troubles, we both felt that subsequent nutritional improvements provided the leading role in her system's ability to cope with the root filled teeth.

In spite of her improvement, she continued to have bouts of ill health from time to time. It is now my opinion that these two root filled teeth should be removed and that she would have been better served had they been extracted in the beginning instead of treated.

Another case, involving a very large cyst, is shown on the x-ray pictures that follow. The cyst looked as though it involved three teeth. We found that the central and lateral incisors were infected; the cuspid tooth was normal and healthy.

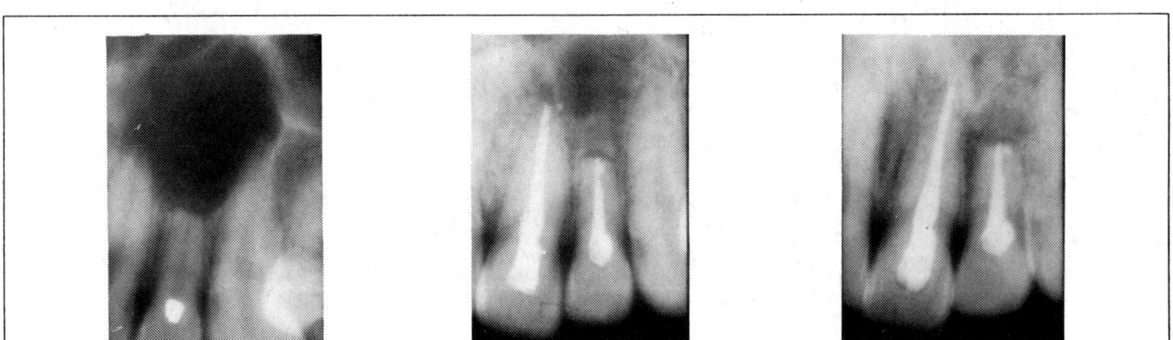

Large cyst from football injury. *6 months post op.* *12 months post op.*

You will note that there are no fillings present in these teeth, meaning that the infection did not come about because of tooth decay; it was felt that the cause in this case was a high school football mouth injury.

Note how small the diameter of the root canal is at the end of the root of the tooth and then visualize an artery, vein, and nerve all entering the tooth at that point. You can readily see how a blow to the mouth or teeth could cause blood vessels to be severed. When that happens, the severed artery cannot heal together fast enough to maintain blood circulation within the tooth.

When a tooth loses its blood supply, the pulp tissue within the root canal dies off for lack of nourishment and gradually rots and putrefies. Eventually it can become infected with bacteria that are present in the blood, and this eventually will cause the eating away of the bone at the end of the tooth's root. In this particular case, the bone of the upper jaw, above the end of the tooth's root, was eaten away clear through the bone at the floor of the nasal cavity.

This young man was a navy pilot flying off a carrier during the Korean War. He wrote to me about having an infected tooth and asked my advice. I suggested he have the ship's navy dentist give him relief and not to permit any extractions.

On his return to the San Diego naval base, he traveled to see me and I performed the apicoectomy surgery and root canal fillings. The two follow-up x-ray pictures were taken at six months and 12 months. You can see the healing was almost complete after one year. After that time the patient moved from the area so I do not have any further follow-ups.

The public should be aware of how difficult it is for a dentist to understand Dr. Price's findings that seemingly healthy teeth are still carrying infection when they see infected holes in jaw bones heal up and stay that way for many years. The thought of bacteria remaining alive in the dentin tubules, mutating, and becoming more virulent and toxic is difficult to comprehend in the face of apparent healing.

Our doubts can only be erased by carefully considering the Dr. Price data regarding the severe illnesses that occurred to thousands of rabbits when diseases were transferred to them from root filled and apicoectomy treated teeth extracted from sick patients.

The reality will become evident when each dentist and each patient tests these findings and experiences their truths. We will then gain an understanding of the mutation versatility of these families of bacteria and their ability to create such havoc for humans and animals.

> *"A new truth is a new sense, for with it comes the ability to see things that we could not see before — and things that cannot be seen by those who do not have that new truth.* – Weston Price

Summary:

- An apicoectomy is an oral surgery root canal treatment procedure that is carried out to save a tooth that might otherwise need to be extracted.

- Even when a large amount of bone has been lost, most of these cases heal uneventfully and new bone is seen to fill in about the end of the root completely in six to 12 months.

- A couple of case histories of apicoectomy surgery from my personal practice are discussed, and before and after x-ray pictures are shown.

- The first of a woman patient is of interest because of large, almost identical granuloma infections showing lateral canals that came from the upper teeth on either side of her two front teeth (lateral incisors). Though her severe gastrointestinal involvement improved dramatically with root canal treatment of these teeth and nutritional counseling, results were not completely satisfactory. With our current knowledge of Dr. Price's research discoveries — and in spite of the long history of service of these two teeth — with hindsight it appears she would have been better served by removal of these teeth.

- The second case involved the largest cyst surgically operated upon, which was caused not by tooth decay but by a football injury. The filling in of new bone at the infection site around the two teeth after six and 12 months proved gratifying to me and the patient. As he moved away, I am unaware of his subsequent health history.

- The successful healing in these two cases emphasizes how difficult it is for dentists and patients alike to believe these teeth could still be carrying infection.

- For those suffering severe degenerative disease problems, it will only be by having seemingly healthy root filled teeth removed that judgement of Price's work will be possible.

- While the percentage of apparent recoveries in such cases is high, it must be kept in mind that other factors can be involved that preclude success.

CHAPTER 20

New Research That Confirms Dr. Price's Discoveries

Because all 1174 pages charting Dr. Price's incredible 25 years of root canal research accomplishments were published back in 1923, there are those who will quickly discount its importance today. Remember, though, that in the history of medicine it is not uncommon for a major advance in thinking to be buried for long periods of time.

The question we should now be asking is: *"What has been learned in the intervening years that confirms Dr. Price's contributions to mankind?"*

Research about endodontic treatment since that time has been extensive and, for the most part, corroborates Dr. Price's discoveries. At the same time, Price's questions go beyond to add new dimensions to understanding problems inherent in the dental profession's effort to save teeth and keep people healthy.

Let me tell you about some of the scientific research that confirms Dr. Price's major revelations and adds so much to our understanding of this subject. What follows includes a bit more technical information than I like to present to lay audiences. However, knowing that some dentists and physicians will read this book because of their own interest in the subject or because of the demands of their patients, it seems necessary to include a minimum of scientific data to emphasize studies that support and confirm the Price discoveries.

The following men made important contributions to society in this regard:

MILTON J. ROSENAU, M.D.

One of the medical greats who contributed much to our knowledge of the process of focal infection was Dr. Milton J. Rosenau, Professor of Preventive Medicine and Hygiene at Harvard Medical School in Boston.

In 1939, in an article published in the *Journal of the American Dental Association*, Rosenau reported isolating streptococci bacteria from an ulcer in the bowel of a patient ill with "mucous colitis." He transferred the bacteria involved in the ulcer through *intravenous* injection to several animals and reproduced in them a similar colitis. Extensive medical work to try and locate the source of the bowel infection was solved when he found the patient had a crowned bicuspid that had a large abscess at its root end.

Cultures made from the infected area were injected intravenously into a rabbit. In 72 hours the rabbit developed a bleeding, necrosing colitis that proved to contain the same family of bacteria involved in the patient's tooth. But Rosenau's experimental work didn't end there. He then planted these bacteria in some of the teeth of a dog. X-ray photographs revealed that these teeth developed abscesses quite similar to that found originally in the patient. What is more, after 16 months the dog developed ulcerative colitis.

To further his work, Dr. Rosenau transferred into the teeth of dogs other strains of streptococci that had been taken from patients with a variety of diseases, either acute or chronic, such as nephritis (kidney disease with stones), cystitis (bladder), stomach ulcers, arthritis, and various central and peripheral nerve diseases. Fifty-two dogs were involved and 1014 dogs who were not inoculated were used as controls. Between 47 percent and 75 percent of the animals developed the same diseases as had the patients.

Dr. Rosenau was criticized that he too often found streptococcus bacteria in diseases transferred via focal infection. He pointed out that the streptococcus organisms were commonly found to be responsible for the largest number of chronic cases of invalidism. You will remember that Dr. Price also found streps the most frequent oral organisms involved in causing degenerative diseases.

FRANK BILLINGS, M.D.

It was Frank Billings, M.D., Dean of the Faculty, Professor and Head of the Department of Medicine and Professor of Medicine at the University of Chicago that located and identified the first focal infection in the mouth. In 1914, Dr. Billings wrote: *"Focal infection is most commonly situated in the head, but may be located in any organ or tissue."* What he meant was, while it was *possible* for a focal infection to arise from anywhere in the body, its most probable starting site was in the mouth.

It must be kept in mind that in the beginning, studies disclosed that the transfer of bacteria from the teeth and tonsils were found to infect the heart, bone joints, kidneys, etc. As time went on, more and more organs and tissues were found to be involved in disease that originated in the mouth.

It would have been better had Dr. Billings been able to spell out the original findings and then to add his new discoveries, for many people who had trouble understanding that bacteria could be transferred from the mouth to other tissues opposed his frequent addition of new areas, even though it should have been obvious that each addition was a new discovery. These objections were partially responsible for the focal infection theory battles that came about.

Eventually Dr. Billings was to state that at least 99 percent of the focally infected diseases arose from the tonsils or teeth, and only one percent or less from all the other sources combined. Some of those other sources proved to be the sinuses, lungs, intestines, toenails, and tonsil tags or stumps, but keep in mind that these bacteria could originate anywhere.

It was Billings who coined the term *focal infection*. Because so many illnesses were chronic streptococcal diseases, such disease involvement became known as the Billings-Rosenau *syndrome*. In a way it is fortunate that the teeth and tonsils are the primary source of these secondary infections, as their accessibility and removal prove a relatively easy solution compared to surgery on major organs.

A strange paradox exists in that a patient who has a severe intestinal or heart problem readily submits to spectacular types of corrective surgery when it would be far simpler and less costly to remove the possible infected tooth, tonsil, or other mouth foci. In Dr. Billings' time, 53 percent of patients who had tonsillectomies required reoperation.

Then too, the dental profession is generally unaware that the first millimeter (less than a sixteenth of an inch) of bone that holds the tooth in its socket can be loaded with bacteria and should be removed at the time of the extraction in order to prevent the trapping of bacteria in the alveolar process, thereby allowing these bony areas to continue to house the organisms. You will find the extraction surgical protocol covered in Chapter 25.

PAUL S. RHOADS, M.D. and GEORGE F. DICK, M.D.

Should you find it difficult to accept that 53 percent of tonsillectomized patients required reoperation, let me add the even more troublesome findings of Drs. Paul S. Rhoads and George F. Dick that appeared in the *Journal of the American Medical Association*: 91, 1149, in 1928. To quote this article directly:

> *"It is shown by this work that tonsillectomy as usually done even by specialists fails to accomplish this end in 73 percent of cases because of incomplete removal of infected tonsillar tissue.*
>
> *...In many instances the condition resulting from incomplete tonsillectomy is worse than that existing before operation.*
>
> *...Patients who had systemic diseases attributable to foci of infection but failed to improve after their original tonsillectomy, improved strikingly after removal of the pieces of tonsillar tissues remaining from the first operation."*

What is so tragic about these surgical failures is that the "stumps" left after tonsillectomy were found to harbor more bacteria per gram than the tonsils that were removed. Assuming that patients were advised to have their tonsils removed because the infected tonsils were causing illness, not removing all the infected tissues accomplished worse than nothing. When these patients then reported that the tonsil removal did not help, they were usually told by the doctor that their illness must be something else. Many of these patients were even accused of being neurotic and were put on drugs for the mentally ill.

Because this study by Drs. Rhoads and Dick was reported in the *A.M.A. Journal* in 1928, we can assume techniques for doing tonsillectomies have improved since then. Those who have undergone this surgery and find that the glands in their neck are still enlarged and perhaps tender, and the tissues about the tonsillectomy scar appear inflamed or are distended, would be wise to consult a surgeon experienced in removing these stumps or tags, as many doctors are not experienced in carefully dissecting out the remaining infected tissue.

It often happens that the patient has two foci of infection present, such as bad tonsils or stumps along with infected teeth. Heart disease, rheumatism, and hyperactivity in the young were seen to arise more frequently from the tonsils, so it proved better to remove them before addressing possibly bad teeth.

Conditions of older people with heart, arthritic, or nerve tissue breakdowns were felt to originate more readily from the teeth. If a child with both dental and tonsil infections had myocarditis, tonsils were removed first, but if the child had endocarditis, priority was given to the removal of the bad teeth.

Ulcers, appendicitis, and muscular rheumatism appeared to be bred most commonly from the softer tonsil tissues.

MELVIN PAGE, D.D.S

Body chemistry health practitioner, Dr. Melvin Page, known for his books *Degeneration—Regeneration, Young Minds With Old Bodies*, and *Your Body is Your Best Doctor*, found that many patients coming to his office had infected tonsil tags. He routinely sent these patients to a surgeon for removal of the tags, as he found it impossible to balance a person's blood chemistry — and particularly their calcium-phosphorus relationship — because of the focal infection they carried. This ties in directly with Price's finding that infections of teeth and gums lowers the amount of calcium in the blood.

Page found support for his findings about tonsil tags in reports by Dr. Otto Meyer of New York City that tonsil tag tissue, even when appearing satisfactory, often contained hidden infection under the scars. Dr. Meyer, in an article in *Eye, Ears, Nose and Throat Monthly*, May 1946, pointed out how veins of the tonsil area also become involved and how the inner walls of a vein can build up and become a new focal infection source. Dr. Meyer's article also covered techniques for removing tonsil tags and inner vein wall infections.

As to the importance of calcium to normal body chemistry activity, Dr. Page was in complete agreement with the Dr. Price findings. All of his work was based upon the calcium-phosphorus balance. In fact, Dr. Page's research carried knowledge of the subject to much greater lengths and advanced understanding. His contribution in this regard was covered in Chapter 11.

The Dr. Melvin Page research concerning the role of the immune system in protecting us from the onslaught of all sources of infection, and how inheritance and nutritional background play a major role in controlling pathogenic organisms, directly confirms Dr. Weston Price's thousands of patient medical history examinations and conclusions.

HAROLD HAWKINS, D.D.S.

It is of much interest that numbers of dental researchers, using entirely different biochemical approaches, have demonstrated the importance of the calcium-phosphorus balance, not only to the development of dental diseases but to that of most other illnesses as well.

In his book, *Applied Nutrition*, Harold Hawkins, D.D.S. showed in his studies of saliva, urine, and feces that Dr. Price was correct when he declared that dental infections reduce the alkalinity of the blood and produce acidosis.

Dr. Hawkins, like Dr. Price, also found that people who had a marked tendency to tooth decay had calcium levels of the saliva and blood that were below normal.

In the case of periodontal disease, Drs. Hawkins and Price seem, on the surface, to be in disagreement with each other. With those not acquainted with the work of both of these men, it must be kept in mind that the studies by Dr. Hawkins' were performed on saliva, urine, and feces, while those of Dr. Price were on blood. In addition, Dr. Price's determinations were based on the amount of ionic calcium present, a figure that can be quite different from that of the *total calcium* in the blood and the saliva.

The loss of bone around teeth having pyorrhea would automatically lead one to believe a low calcium condition was present, but Dr. Price found such cases had high amounts of ionic calcium. Hawkins, on the other hand, found that most people with periodontal disease had low amounts of calcium in their saliva and high phosphorus. Less commonly, he found some cases had low calcium/low phosphorus balances. Very occasionally he found a third type that had high calcium and low phosphorus readings in their saliva.

In reviewing the considerable amount of research that has taken place in the field of *endodontia*, scientific literature contains many reports that substantiate the Price studies. A few will be included now, as their data will further help to dispel any notion that Dr. Price's disclosures in 1923 were not true discoveries.

MAX WINSLOW, D.D.S. and SAMUEL H. MILLSTONE, B.S., D.D.S

This first report comes from the Dental Division of the Sinai Hospital in Detroit, Michigan, by Drs. Winslow and Millstone that was published in the *Journal of Periodontal Research*, September and October 1965. It concerns the bacteremia that occurs in all people after routine prophylaxis (tooth cleaning) by their dentist or hygienist. It has been well-established that any dental procedures that are accompanied by bleeding allow bacteria present in the mouth to readily enter into the bloodstream.

Such bacteremias are usually of short duration and are of no threat to the patient. However, those who have had rheumatic heart disease or other heart problems are at more risk of attracting these bacteria to their deformed or damaged heart valves.

The doctors reported that about 20 percent of people with heart problems who have dental procedures develop bacterial endocarditis within several weeks of their prophylaxis appointment. As mentioned in an earlier chapter, the American Heart Association and medical profession require that dentists prescribe antibiotics for certain heart patients both before and after any dental treatment to prevent the occurrence of such focal infections.

It was also pointed out that the routine use of antibiotics as standard practice has resulted in the development of resistant strains of bacteria, not to mention the side effects the drugs produce. Dr. Price's finding that bacteria remaining in root filled teeth became very resistant to disinfectants and even more virulent was laughed at. And what is worse is that he was accused of fabricating the information.

Drs. Winslow and Millstone also tested the use of topical iodine germicides and reported that there was a significant reduction in bacteremia when germicides were applied to gums and teeth before dental treatment. Further studies by others about the use of preoperative medicaments will be covered in the reports that follow.

E. CHERASKIN, M.D., D.M.D., M.A. and W. RINGSDORF, Jr., D.M.D., M.S.
Among the numerous blood study changes experienced by patients having root canal fillings was that of an upset carbohydrate metabolism. Dr. Price found this was accompanied by increased amounts of sugar in their blood (hyperglycemia) and in the urine (glycosuria). Doctors Cheraskin and Ringsdorf reported in four articles appearing in the *Journal of Oral Medicine,* January, April and July of 1968 and November of 1987, that though the numbers tested (55) was small, there was statistically significant evidence of a disturbance of carbohydrate metabolism among endodontic patients.

MERVIN D. KLOTZ, D.D.S, M.S.; HAROLD GERSTEIN, D.D.S. and ARTHUR N. BOHN, Ph.D.

Twenty-four infected teeth in five monkeys were tested for the occurrence of bacteremia after prednisolone powder (a corticosteriod) was placed over pulps exposed by tooth decay. The procedures were confined to the pulp chamber and did not extend near the root apex or beyond.

Of the 19 trials in which prednisolone was used to treat infected pulps, four (21 percent) developed bacteremia. The four trials that resulted in the presence of bacteremia in the blood represented 36 percent of the total. If only one of the 19 tested caused a bacteremia after corticosteriod placement, the result would have been significant as virulent organisms can cause serious damage to the body.

Because of the risk of endocarditis or serious heart and other tissue problems, dentists who use corticosteroids should also be using antibiotics to try and control the effects of a likely secondary focal infection. It is prednisolone's action in *preventing* the phagocytosis destruction of organisms that increases the risk of bacteremia. Lay readers should be aware that the amount of steroids used inside a tooth on a pulp exposure is miniscule, yet it is able to significantly increase the number of bacteria invading the bloodstream.

AKE MOLLAR, J.R.

Bacteriologic studies that have taken place since the Price research about various kinds of bacteria has added much to our knowledge. Almost all of these studies have concerned the bacteria present in root canals, but almost no work has been done about those present in dentin tubules.

In one recent study concerning the presence of bacteria in dentin tubules preceding the advancement of dental caries, it was found that the pulp in the pulp chamber undergoes inflammatory changes before a visible exposure is made by the tooth decay process. Dr. Price not only pointed this out, he published pictures demonstrating the early presence of pulp inflammation in Chapter 17 of his first volume about dental infections.

An exceptionally thorough book, *Root Canals and Periapical Tissues of Human Teeth,* by Ake Mollar of the Department of Bacteriology, University of Gotenburg and the Department of Cardiology and Endodontology, University of Lund in Sweden, published in 1966, details many new groups of bacteria that have been isolated and divides them into four groups. Like Dr. Price, Dr. Mollar found the organisms most frequently present were of the streptococcus viridans group.

Of significant concern to Price were several common beliefs of fellow dentists, including: the ready acceptance of dentists to trust the appearance of a root canal filled tooth on x-ray pictures to determine whether it was still infected; and to consider a tooth still infected only if pus, drainage, or an offensive smell was present. Here too, Dr. Mollar and Dr. Price were in agreement. Dr. Mollar listed the reports of 15 researchers who also felt a proper diagnosis had to be based upon microbiological methods to establish if the root canal had been made sterile.

GORA SUNDQUIST

In 1976, Gora Sundquist and the UMEA University in Sweden published the *Odontological Dissertations No. 7* monograph under the title, "Bacteriologic Studies of Necrotic Dental Pulps."

Sundquist reported that anaerobic (ability to live without need of oxygen) bacteria made up from 24 to 32 percent of the bacteria strains they found in teeth and that many strains found in root canals had not previously been described.

Surprisingly, most species found in pulp chambers are the same ones present in the gum crevices about each tooth. Three of these species are not found in high numbers in other parts of the mouth. Sundquist stated that these bacteria could travel to the pulp chamber by way of dentin tubules but could also get there indirectly by being absorbed into the bloodstream, eventually ending up in the pulp chamber via the artery coming into the root end of the tooth.

Price demonstrated how bacteria in periodontal pockets were absorbed into the tooth through any lateral canals that opened into the area of the pyorrhea pocket, as well as through the dentin tubules.

S.L. BAHN; D. ROSS; T. BIENCEVENGA and A.H. BAHN

Some critics of the Price research regarding the development of endocarditis from dental sources have claimed the evidence to be circumstantial. However, experimental studies have proven, without a doubt, a direct causal relationship. One study, by Drs. Bahn, Ross, Biencevenga, and Bahn, and carried out at the West Haven Veterans Hospital in Connecticut, and S.I.U., Edwardsville, Illinois, appeared in an article in the *Journal of Dental Research*, Special Issue, Volume 53, February 1974.

Surgically, the investigators introduced vegetative infected lesions directly on the heart valves of albino rabbits by placing sterile polyethylene catheters into their heart valves. They were then able to introduce and challenge the animals with the bacteria strain streptococcus mutants or streptococcus mitis which had been isolated and cultured from humans who had endocarditis. These bacteria were introduced by intravenous injection into a rabbit's ear vein and into the socket of an extracted incisor, or into gum tissue.

Four out of five animals inoculated with strep mitis injected into the ear developed vegetation growths. The catheter route produced infected heart valves in all 12 animals challenged with the strep mitis, and all 12 challenged with strep mutants. None of the control animals developed lesions. All of the animals receiving strep mitis survived the first week, while the mortality rate of the second group receiving strep mutants was 50 percent. Only three of 18 rabbits that received the bacteria in the tooth socket or gums developed heart valve lesions.

The introduction of viable streptococcus mitis and mutans by the insertion of polyethyline catheters into the aortic valves of rabbits predisposed to infection produced lesions that were histologically similar to those observed in human endocarditis.

D.A. McGOWAN, M.D.S., F.D.S., F.F.D. and J.M. HARDIE, B.D.S., L.D.S., DIP. BACT.

The work of these scientists was carried out in the departments of Bacteriology and Oral Surgery of the Dental School at the London Hospital Medical College and was reported in the *British Dental Journal*, Vol. 137 (No. 4), August 20, 1974.

Their research involving 20 rabbits produced lesions in the animals' hearts by introducing streptococcus bacteria through a polyethylene cannula that was inserted in the heart. In this study, bacteria that were involved in deposits scaled from the teeth and gum crevices of the animals were used.

No organisms were found in the five control animals. All of the other rabbits developed visible signs of heart lesions. From three of these rabbits, Dr. McGowan and Hardie were able to identify and grow bacteria found in the lesions. These experiments proved without a doubt that bacterial endocarditis did not arise accidentally but occurred as a direct result of dental treatment.

In their report, these two British doctors listed the names of many scientists and physicians investigating the various aspects of transference of oral organisms to other body tissues. Just in case there are any more doubting Thomas' out there, the list below gives the names of those who confirmed the relationship that exists between bacteremia arising from dental treatment and the occurrence of bacterial endocarditis in susceptible patients.

These scientists are: Ruston (1930); Garrod and Waterworth (1962); Archard and Roberts (1966); Jokinen (1970); Carlsson (1967); de Stoppelaar (1971); White and Niven (1946); Hehre (1948); Porterfield (1950); and Farmer (1953).

While I am most pleased to be able to reproduce this list of individuals who substantiated key phases of the Dr. Price research, it is surprising that Drs. McGowan and Hardie did not include the name of Dr. Price himself and Drs. Billings, Rosenau, Truman, Brophy, Ladd, Garrey, Vaughn, Welch, Hektoen, and Charles Mayo who were so important to this work in the 1920s, 30s, and 40s. This appears to be additional evidence of how successful the anti-focal infection groups were in silencing the work of these great men.

I.B. BENDER, D.D.S. and STEVE MONTGOMERY, D.D.S

Dr. Bender has been one of the great contributors to the advancement of endodontia. His 1986 article, written in conjunction with Dr. Montgomery,

"Non-Surgical Endodontic Procedure for the Patient at Risk for Infective Endocarditis and Other Systemic Disorders," published in the *Journal of Endodontics*, Volume 12, No. 9, September 1986, was among more than 50 articles I reviewed in trying to bring the Price information up-to-date.

It proved to be the most outstanding for everyday practical use by dentists and patients by showing how they can combat the focal infection dangers of heart and joint risk conditions.

Drs. Bender and Montgomery stated that the American Heart Association, in publishing their guidelines regarding the reduction of bacteremia, reinforced the fact that any bleeding in the mouth contributed to bacterial contamination of the blood. However, the A.H.A. did not provide any guidelines for non-surgical, everyday endodontic treatment, or the daily home care needs of these patients.

Bender pointed out that evidence regarding non-surgical procedures of cleaning, reaming, and filling root canals produced no detectable bacteremias unless vigorous instrumentation was carried out through the root end of the tooth into the surrounding bony area of the jaw.

When such vigorous instrumentation occurred, detectable bacteremia took place in 15 of 48 cases (31.2 percent). It was felt that the routine placement of the rubber dam clamp could produce some bleeding, particularly in mouths in which oral hygiene practices were poor. However, the amount of bacteria introduced would be small and could be controlled with the use of topical de-germing disinfectants.

Bender and Montgomery's examination of a variety of de-germing procedures resulted in their testing and tabulating the results of preparations made by eight dentists. Their tests of the eight different disinfectants involved some 857 patients. The only disinfectant that completely prevented any bacteremia was one composed of iodine and glycerine. A 0.2 percent chlorhexidine mouth rinse having an 87 percent success rate in controlling bacteremia proved the most efficient mouthwash.

Before penicillin, there was an almost 100 percent fatality rate in infective endocarditis cases. Although antibiotics have been responsible for the 70 to 90 percent reduction of deaths in such cases, there has *not* been any increase in the reduction of their numbers since the start of the penicillin era. There has been a reduction in the number of young people with infected hearts, but that has been due to the decrease in the occurrence of rheumatic heart disease.

On the other hand, there has been an increase in the number of heart complications occurring in older patients. Dr. Bender points out that there has been a change in the types of streptococcus organisms involved in these heart conditions and that occasionally streptococcus fecalis from the oral cavity and root canals have been isolated.

This is of interest as strep fecalis was the strain of streptococcus that Price found most prevalent, being present 65 $^{1}/_{2}$ percent of the time. However, while fecalis was involved in only three percent of the Dr. Price heart cases, this streptococcus strain was involved in 21 percent of cases that involved nerves, and to a somewhat lessor extent in rheumatism and diseases involving other tissues and organs.

The two charts that follow appeared in an early chapter. They tabulate the bacteria Dr. Price isolated and the diseases they caused. The repetition here will allow your comparison with more current findings.

RELATIVE PREVALENCE OF DIFFERENT STRAINS

*Type of Streptococcus	%	Graphic Expressions
Fecalis	65½	
Ignavius	1½	
Salivarius	1½	
Infrequens	9	
Mitis	7½	
Non-Hemolyticus I	3	
Non-Hemolyticus III	3	
Hemolyticus I	3	
Subacidus	1½	
Pyogenes	4½	

Type of Lesion in Patient	S. Ignavius	S. Salivarius	S. Infrequens	S. Mitis	S. Non-Hemolyticus I	S. Non-Hemolyticus III	S. Hemolyticus I	S. Subacidus	S. Pyogenes	S. Fecalis	Percentage S. Fecalis	Ratio of Chance
Rheumatism			2		1	1				**7**	11	**7.1**
Heart										**2**	3	**1.3**
Nerves		1	3	4	2	1	2		3	**21**	33	**24.05**
Lassitude			2	1						**11**	17	**9.1**
Internal Organs		1	1	1						**8**	13	**7.1**
Special Tissues	1		3	1		3				**7**	11	**9 7**
No Lesions								1		**7**	11	**5.2**

It is clear that patients at risk of developing bacterial endocarditis and their dentists should be following a much more inclusive prevention program than just the use of an antibiotic. Scrupulous home hygiene practices including the use of home care disinfectants or mouth rinses of proven bactericidal efficacy must be adopted. In addition, the use of topical degerming agents by the dentist or hygienist is essential before any dental procedures are undertaken.

It is shocking that physicians and dentists seldom investigate the possible presence of other focal infection sources as part of their preoperative bacterial endocarditis prevention programs. Patients must be examined to determine the presence of any infected teeth, gums, tonsil tags, or other possible sources of focal infection. Then too, in view of Dr. Price's work, patients should be queried about any past root canal treated teeth as they may not only be a factor in the current disease problem but could actually be a cause of it.

Martin H. Fischer, M.D., a prolific writer of medical books during the 1940s, had this to say:

> *"Focal infection started in a tooth is obviously no trivial matter! From it are destined to flow into the periphery (other glands, organs and tissues) what amounts to unexpected and acute or chronic invalidism at the best; at the worst, death."*

Perhaps now we can truly evaluate how unfortunate it was that the Dr. Price research was covered-up and buried all these years. When you think of all the excellent research accomplished by those mentioned in this chapter, it might lead you to think that this subject is now clarified and out in the open. However, the fact is that only a handful of dentists in the country have any knowledge about the Dr. Weston Price work. Although recent studies have been published in scientific journals, I dare say that very few dentists or physicians in the country have read or know anything about their content.

Of course, both dentists and physicians are very familiar with the risks causing endocarditis by way of dental treatment, but for most health professionals this book will probably be their first introduction to the phenomenal extent of the focal infection problem.

Summary:

- It has not been uncommon in the history of medicine for a major advance in the cure of disease to be buried for long periods of time as a result of controversy.

- When the theories behind a research endeavor become "dated," the inevitable question arises as to what follow-up studies have confirmed the original premise. In Dr. Price's case there have been many; since 15 key studies are listed.

- *Dr. Milton I. Rosenau, Professor of Preventive Medicine, Harvard Medical School*. Dr. Rosenau did many experiments using dogs and other animals.

A good example was transferring the ulcerative colitis of a patient to several kinds of animals. Colleagues at the time criticized his finding streptococcus the most common bacteria involved in degenerative diseases but it confirmed Dr. Price's discoveries and still holds true today.

- *Frank Billings, M.D., Dean of the Faculty, Professor and Head of Department of Medicine, University of Chicago.* Dr. Billings was the person who identified the first occurrence of focal infection arising from the mouth. He was eventually able to determine that 99 percent of focally infected diseases arose in the mouth from the teeth and the tonsils. He found the other one percent could come from any tissue, but most often involved the sinuses, lungs, intestines, toenails, and tonsil tags or stumps.

  It was Dr. Billings who named this process "focal infection." Even during his time, it was common for people suffering degenerative disease problems to have the gland or organ surgically removed. The paradox is that patients are willing to submit to severe surgical procedures but, at the same time, are reluctant to remove an infected tooth. Obviously, tooth removal would be far simpler, less traumatic and less costly. Patients, for the most part, come to the conclusion to have surgery because their doctors do not present this alternative, nor do their dentists.

- *Paul S. Rhoads, M.D.; George F. Dick, M.D.* These two physicians in an article in the *American Medical Association Journal* in 1928 reported finding 73 percent of tonsillectomies, even those done by specialists, failed to remove all the tonsillar tissue. They found this resulted in infective conditions that were worse than those that existed before the tonsillectomy.

  Many patients who had tonsils removed as a focal infection source failed to improve, but strikingly did so after the tags or stumps were thoroughly excised.

  As this study took place so long ago, it might be assumed that tonsillectomies are better performed today. However, those who have had tonsils removed and are experiencing enlarged, tender or sore glands in their neck or inflamed stumps should consult a physician who follows the specialized technique of removing these infected areas.

- *Melvin Page, D.D.S.* A body chemistry practitioner, Dr. Page found he could not balance a patient's chemistry if a tonsil tag remained. Some of his knowledge grew out of his contacts with Dr. Otto Meyer of New York City who, in an article appearing in the *Eye, Ears, Nose and Throat*

Monthly, May 1946, pointed out how veins in tonsils can build up with bacteria and become a new focal infection source. His article covered specialized techniques that proved helpful in removing these inner throat wall infections.

Dr. Page found that a patient's calcium/phosphorus balance was the key to solving their degenerative disease problems. When balance of these two elements was achieved, illnesses miraculously disappeared. His work confirms Dr. Price's findings about the importance of calcium. The titles of Dr. Page's three books are contained in this chapter.

- *Harold Hawkins, D.D.S.* Dr. Hawkins' research was much like that of Dr. Price's. However, his studies didn't concern blood but rather concentrated on saliva, urine, feces, and the acid-base balance.

  Dr. Hawkins was a dentist with a chemistry laboratory but not a dental chair. Many of his discoveries paralleled those of Dr. Price, but some of his calcium conclusions appear different because Dr. Price investigated ionic calcium values while Dr. Hawkins investigated total calcium.

  Like Drs. Page and Price, Dr. Hawkins based much of what appears in his outstanding book, *Applied Nutrition*, on the calcium-phosphorus balance. His case history records involving 10,000 patients showed a remarkable ability to arrest dental caries and periodontal disease by nutritional means.

- *Max Winslow, D.D.S. and Samuel H. Millstone, B.S., D.D.S. from the dental division of the Sinai Hospital in Detroit.* These doctors found that bactermia from dental care was usually of short duration, but that 20 percent of people with heart problems did develop bacterial endocarditis within several weeks of routine prophylaxis (tooth cleaning).

  This is, of course, another demonstration of the focal infection theory in action. While Dr. Price was laughed at for his similar pronouncements, these two doctors have been praised.

- *E. Cheraskin, M.D., D.M.D., M.A.; W.M. Ringsdorf, Jr., D.M.D., M.S.* Reported in four articles in *Journal of Oral Medicine* 1968 - 1987 evidence of disturbed carbohydrate metabolism among endodontic treated patients, confirming Dr. Price's finding of increased amounts of sugar in blood and urine of these patients.

- *Mervin D. Klotz, D.D.S., M.S.; Harold Gerstein, D.D.S.; Arthur N. Bohn, Ph.D.* In testing tiny, miniscule amounts of prednisilone (a corticosteroid) over exposed nerves in the teeth of five monkeys, they found 21 percent developed bacteremia. This indicates a need for antibiotics when steroids are used.

- *Ake Mollar, J.R.*, working in the Department of Bacteriology, University of Gotenburg, and the Department of Cardiology and Endodontology, University of Lund in Sweden found many new groups of bacteria but concluded in his 1966 book that the most frequent one present was the streptococcus viridans group, the same one Dr. Price discovered years before.

  Dr. Mollar pointed out that the pulp of the tooth was found to develop inflammation before tooth decay was visible. Dr. Price showed a picture of this phenomenon in his 1923 publications yet few dentists are aware even today of this important point.

  Like Dr. Price, Dr. Mollar expressed concern regarding the average dentist's acceptance and trust of the appearance of a root filled tooth on an x-ray picture as to whether or not an infection was present. Regarding whether or not a root canal had been made sterile, Mollar and 15 other researchers made the statement that a proper diagnosis must be based on microbiological methods.

  Dr. Mollar did not mention dentin tubule infection but all his research strongly supports the Weston Price findings.

- *Gora Sundquist.* With improved techniques for isolating bacteria, Sundquist, in 1974 and 1975 at the UMAE University in Sweden, was able to isolate 88 strains of bacteria, many of which had not been described or found in root canals previously and only five of which grew in the presence of air.

  His assertions that bacteria could travel to the pulp chamber by way of the dentin tubules was also pointed out by Dr. Price, but Dr. Sundquist's claim that bacteria could be picked up by the bloodstream, circulate through the body, and be introduced inside of the tooth through its blood supply entering at the roots' apex, is a whole new concept.

- *S.L. Bahn; D. Ross; T. Biencevenga; A.H. Bahn.* Some have claimed the development of heart cases from dental sources to be circumstantial. However, this team of investigators introduced infective lesions directly into heart valves of rabbits using catheters. Thereafter, they were able to challenge the animals in a number of different ways, proving heart lesions could arise from dental infections.

- *D.A. McGowan, M.D.S., F.D.S., F.F.D.; J.M. Hardie, B.D.S., L.D.S., DIP. BACT.* These London researchers of the Bacteriology and Oral Surgery Department of the Dental School at the London Hospital Medical College also proved that streptococcus bacteria from gum crevices and deposits scaled from teeth when introduced via a cannula inserted into the heart of 20 rabbits definitely produced visible heart lesions in all but the five control animals. They thereby proved that bacterial endocarditis can occur as a direct result of dental treatment.

  The McGowan group, expecting some would doubt endocarditis could be introduced by bacteremia due to dental treatment, tested the work of 13 scientists whose reports grace scientific literature supporting this view. I added an additional 11 names that they had missed; for their identity, see the McGowan data in this chapter.

- *I.B. Bender, D.D.S.; Steve Montgomery, D.D.S.* In a 1986 article, the authors point out the great increase in heart complications occurring in older patients. They confirm that the streptococcus fecalis family Dr. Price found prevaled 65.5 percent of the time was the predominant one that were inhabiting the oral cavity and root canals.

  Another extremely important contribution of Drs. Bender and Montgomery was their review of the inadequacies of antibiotics in controlling bacteremia from the mouth because of the tremendous number of bacteria involved therein.

  Whereas antibiotics control relatively few species of bacteria, they found that in studies of eight dentists involving 857 patients that a topical degerming — using a solution of iodine in glycerine — was 100 percent effective in controlling bacteremia. Furthermore, they listed a mouthwash (0.2 percent chlorhexidine) as having an 87 percent success rate in controlling bacteremia.

  In view of the numbers of bacterial endocarditis heart cases that developed two to three weeks after dental treatment, it behooves the dental and medical professions to promote degerming procedures and to investigate other potential foci that may be present.

This information of Dr. Bender, one of the country's leading endodontists, gives me hope that the American Association of Endodontists will address these focal infection problems as quickly as possible.

- There has been such confidence placed in the use of antibiotics by physicians and dentists that they rarely think to examine people's mouths for obvious gum or tooth infections, infected tonsils, tonsil tags, etc. Very few dentists or other health professionals have the slightest inkling as to the potential dangers of hidden mouth infections, especially in root canal filled teeth.

  This book for most will be their introduction into the side effects inherent in a root canal filled tooth.

- *Martin H. Fischer, M.D.* A professor of physiology and prolific writer of medical books. In 1940 he pointed out that focal infection arising from a tooth is no trivial matter, and that germs easily flow from the mouth to other glands and organs, resulting in acute or chronic invalidism at best; at worst death.

  You can readily see that research by outstanding professionals since Dr. Price's time substantiates his basic discoveries.

  In spite of all that has been revealed in leading professional publications no one has come forth to bring this noteworthy information to the public.

CHAPTER 21

The 30 Rabbits Study

Getting Results Comparable to Double Blind Studies

Most of the information in this chapter has been presented elsewhere throughout this book. It is being repeated here, altogether, in order to counter criticisms that Dr. Price's studies were devoid of double blind studies — and that his work is anecdotal, that is, a figure of his own personal prejudices and imagination.

Though double blind studies where unknown in Dr. Price's time, he was personally aware of how easy it was to allow personal beliefs to creep into any scientific investigations.

The purpose of bringing all this particular information back into one chapter is to emphasize and demonstrate the numbers of ways Dr. Price carried out his research to avoid misinterpretation.

The sheer repeating of the various tests and the great variety of methods used accentuates the thoroughness and importance of his efforts.

For example, in order to determine whether the reactions that occurred to teeth when they were placed under the skin of rabbits were caused by the irritation of their presence or were due to the action of bacteria, a number of tests were devised.

One mentioned earlier was the placement of sterile objects under the skins of rabbits. It did not matter whether a coin, a piece of sterile glass, or any one of a number of ordinary metals was placed under a rabbit's skin, little change took place about any of these foreign bodies except for the formation of a cyst-like covering that was always found to be sterile. You will note that the picture of a dime on page 4 that was inserted under a rabbit's skin shows that the inscription could clearly be read through the thin cystic capsule.

When healthy teeth free from infection, such as freshly extracted impacted wisdom teeth or decay free bicuspids removed for orthodontic purposes, were implanted under the skin of a rabbit or in muscle tissue, no reaction whatever was seen; no matter how long they were left imbedded, the rabbits lived full and healthy lives. At the time the picture showing the coin was taken, two months had elapsed. *Over 100 of these tests using foreign objects were made to verify this finding.*

A very great difference occurred to animals when teeth containing root canal fillings were embedded. Some of these imbedded teeth developed a closely adherent, fibrous capsule around them that was quite different than the cystic sac around the dime. When no capsule formed, the embedded tooth was found to be surrounded by a well of inflamed exudate liquid or pus, and sometimes the area was filled with leucocytes (white blood cells that destroy bacteria). At times none of these protective cells were present, but many streptococcus bacteria would be found.

When no capsule was formed, the rabbits usually died in from a day and a half to a few weeks, but most often in six days. When these teeth became surrounded by a capsule, the rabbits generally lived for several months to a year and, in many instances, they didn't show the slightest evidence of any injury from the presence of the teeth.

Others that were completely encapsulated didn't show any signs of injury or abscessing for weeks, but the animals would quite often develop degenerative diseases of the heart and kidneys. When a rabbit built a capsule about the infected tooth, the capsule invariably began to absorb the tooth in an effort to get rid of it.

One of Dr. Price's critics claimed humans were usually able to control the infection of teeth without dying, but a rabbit, being only one twentieth the size of a human, would be overwhelmed. In order to test that supposition, after a rabbit would die of an implanted tooth, Price retrieved the tooth, cleansed and washed it with pumice, and implanted it again in another rabbit. Thereafter, a total of 30 rabbits had that same tooth quickly re-implanted after the death of its predecessor.

It was determined that the toxins produced by the bacteria, not the bacteria themselves, killed the rabbits and it was supposed that the toxic substances in the tooth would gradually diminish with each implantation. The actual amount of poison in a single tooth isn't very great, so it was expected to be completely gone after 20 rabbits had been used. It was also assumed that with each succeeding rabbit, that rabbit's life span would become longer than the first rabbit's as the poisons dissipated. Instead, they all died within six days, except for one that lived 10 days.

This particular rabbit was a very large and vigorous male and an ugly fighter that tried to kill others in the cage. Within six hours of the tooth implantation, it lost all of its pugnacity and viciousness. In a couple of days, blood changes such as the reduction of ionic calcium appeared and the rabbit began to lose weight.

Calcium values of the animals that developed capsulations about the embedded teeth tended to stay the same, while in others the calcium progressively became less and less, and in some it dropped to zero. Whenever a rabbit failed to build an encapsulating membrane, it would die quickly. In other words, the encapsulation provided some degree of temporary immunity.

It may prove difficult for the average person to comprehend the concept that these deaths are *not* being caused by bacteria but by the poisons or toxins they produce. To demonstrate that these infirmities can be due to toxins, Price crushed the roots of root filled teeth, washed them, and passed the washings through a Berkefeld filter, a method that removes all bacteria. Culturing the remaining solution to see if any bacteria had been retained proved that none were. Nevertheless, that remaining liquid, when it was inoculated into rabbits, would start their decline. In addition, there occurred a depression of their normal ionic calcium level, a progressive loss of weight, and death usually resulted in a few weeks.

These facts suggested the encapsulating sack is not a typical neoplasm (tumor) but is a protective membrane developed by nature to protect the animal carrying it. What occurs appears to be a defense mechanism to save the rabbit, but in these cases it can do so only temporarily because of the virulence of the toxins that are continually being produced by the bacteria in the dentin tubules.

Of all of the experiments Price did with rabbits, the most surprising results occurred when he removed an infected tooth that had been embedded in a rabbit that had died and then placed it in boiling water for one hour. When the tooth cooled off, it was re-embedded in another rabbit. An encapsulation took place and in about two weeks blood changes started to occur which resulted in that rabbit dying in a period of 22 days.

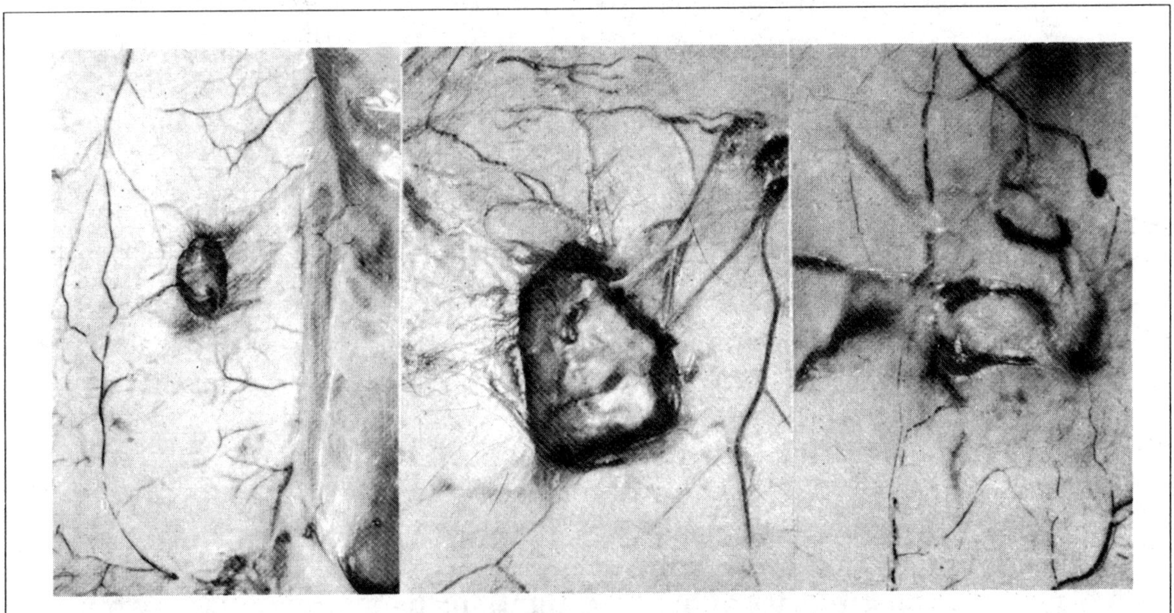

Encapsulations about boiled infected teeth. Heating did not destroy the toxins.

In a similar experiment, the infected tooth was subjected to heat and 30 pounds pressure for one hour in a hospital autoclave sterilizer normally used to sterilize instruments. After the tooth was placed under the skin of a rabbit, the rabbit lost 31 percent of its weight and, being obviously near death, was put to sleep with chloroform.

Then in another test, a tooth that previously had been implanted in several rabbits in succession resulting in their deaths was autoclaved at 60 pounds pressure for one hour. One would think the rabbit would be unaffected in this case, but though it lived longer, it too died in 35 days after losing 36 pounds of its normal weight.

Still Dr. Price wasn't satisfied that these tests were proof enough so he autoclaved some additional root filled teeth at an incredible 300 pounds pressure and this time for two hours. Then in some other cases, infected teeth were placed in very strong chemical disinfectants. In both groups, the teeth developed encapsulation tissue, a type of tissue sack about them. Even so, blood changes took place and these rabbits were also unable to survive.

One would believe that such sterilization procedures would kill bacteria in these teeth and make them as safe as natural, healthy ones, but even if the organisms themselves died, there were apparently sufficient toxins remaining that the animals became ill and died. Although double blind studies were not heard of in Dr. Price's time, he was very conscious of the problems involved in accepting anecdotal test results. That is the reason he repeated test procedures so often in so great a number of different ways, and why he found it necessary to use so many rabbits. All of his investigations were designed to rule out mistaken interpretations.

Numbers of times Price stated that he felt confident that his interpretations were sound and factual but, at the same time, he encouraged future investigators to test his findings. He, above all things, wanted — and worked for — truth to prevail.

Summary:

- There is no question that most scientists today will be skeptical of the Dr. Price research, claiming his results to be anecdotal — that his reports and stories are derived from his own personal beliefs and prejudices.

- Double blind studies, designed to prevent such misinterpretaions, were not known or used at the time of the Price research.

- Although Dr. Price knew nothing of such procedures, he was acutely aware of the possibilities of his investigations being influenced by his own feelings and past experiences.

- It was his consciousness of such a possibility that led to his repeating studies so many times, in so many different ways, and using so many animals.

- For example, when a rabbit became ill and died of a specific illness, he would replant the same tooth in numbers of other animals to verify whether or not the same illness would be repeated.

- With several types of infections, he transferred the patient's tooth into 30 rabbits, and in one series of experiments he repeated the process in 100 animals. In all instances, the disease being investigated reoccurred.

- It was pointed out in this chapter that when healthy teeth extracted for orthodontic purposes or impacted wisdom teeth were implanted, nothing harmful happened to the rabbits. Implanted sterile coins, glass and other items produced no harm to the animals. These tests were carried out 100 times to rule out possible error.

- The most startling study was one in which an infected tooth was removed from a rabbit that had died of a patient's illness. In this case, the tooth was washed and pumiced and then placed in boiling water for one hour. This tooth, when imbedded in another rabbit, resulted in the rabbit dying in 22 days.

- Even more amazing was an even more stringent investigation. Teeth that had been implanted in rabbits several times, causing illness and death, were subjected to hospital autoclave temperatures and pressures of 30 pounds and 60 pounds for one hour. An additional test was carried out at 300 pounds pressure for 2 hours. Still, when those teeth were imbedded in rabbits, the animals lost weight, developed blood changes and died — not as rapidly, but in 35 days.

- Studies were undertaken to determine if the deaths were occurring because of infection from bacteria. In these studies, root filled teeth were crushed, washed, and the washings were passed through a Berkefeld filter — a method that removes all bacteria. The remaining solution was then subjected to culturing to prove all bacteria had been successfully removed from the solution. When this solution was inoculated into rabbits, it caused them to decline; their ionic calcium was lowered, loss of weight took place, and death occurred in a few weeks.

- These experiments demonstrated that the toxins of the bacteria were more lethal than the direct action of bacteria.

- Even though Price felt confident that his research and interpretations were sound and factual, he encouraged future investigators to further test his findings.

To Dr. Price, the uncovering of truth was the most important objective of his research. He hoped that the future would shed more light on his studies — and take them further. That his deductions would be ultimately proved or disproved was of little concern. What was of concern was that truth be found.

CHAPTER 22

Death and Dentistry

"Like the metastasis of cancer, microorganisms from teeth and tonsils metastasize to other organs and result in similar circumstances."

– E.C. Rosenow, M.D.

* * *

"In their addiction to the slogan 'save the tooth' dentists increasingly lose the patient."

– M.H. Fisher, M.D.

* * *

The title of Dr. Fischer's book, *Death and Dentistry*, and the above statement by Dr. E.C. Rosenow, M.D. may hit dentists and patients like a hard blow to the pit of the stomach. Somehow, when Dr. Price said the members of the dental profession are going to have to face up and reassess their role in the cause of the tremendous increase of degenerative diseases, we never thought of these afflictions as causing death but merely as being treatable illnesses.

Now here comes a physician who writes a book about teeth entitled *Death and Dentistry*, published in 1940, seventeen years after Dr. Price's two books, urging the dental profession to wake up. He points out how many of our patients develop endocarditis, a chronic appendix, or a bleeding ulcer and often end up with their illness worsening and their immune system shot — or perhaps they develop another disease such as pneumonia, and in time they may even die as the result of a focal infection.

Most surgeries that are performed for various degenerative conditions involve the amputation of some body part. Sure these operations usually stop the immediate pain, arrest the progress of the disease temporarily, and lengthen life for a while. When such diseases occur, people are willing to submit to a surgical removal of one of their body parts for relief when it would make more sense to remove the focal infected tooth or tonsils causing all the trouble. After all, teeth are easily accessible, are relatively safe to remove, heal quickly, and extraction is a much more cost efficient operation.

The dental profession and dentists generally have been noted for their long history of educating people about the benefits of saving their teeth and preventing dental disease. For the most part, we can say that dentists today believe in the focal infection theory — that is, that teeth can harbor infection that can be transferred to other organs or tissues. Most practicing dentists have had patients that were cured of a medical problem when an oral infection was removed.

What we haven't known all these years, and fail even today to recognize, is the extent to which root canal filled teeth can continue to harbor infection when they seemingly appear to have been successfully treated.

Worse than that is how few dentists have any knowledge of the hidden side effects of root canal fillings, how they occur, and why they are responsible for an infinite variety of serious degenerative diseases that ravage our bodies. Needless to say, none of us have been fully aware of the connection between these occurrences and the number of people who die because of them.

Generally, the average dentist in all of his or her years of practice is not aware of any patient dying as a result of dental treatment. Of all my dentist acquaintances, I do not know of a single one who has knowingly lost a patient.

Suddenly, as a result of these numerous studies by numbers of authorities, we must look at our role in the instigation of endocarditis, kidney or liver disease, and all of the other possible focal infection illnesses that debilitate and encourage susceptibility to other illnesses. How many people are dying before their time because of hidden polymorphic bacteria?

For a physician to write about teeth and their relationship to illness and death is a most unusual and rare confirmation of the Dr. Weston Price work. However, Dr. Fischer was well-qualified to write about this subject for physicians as he was Professor of Physiology at the University of Cincinnati, authored eight medical books on a variety of subjects, and translated five additional books of foreign publishers.

Earlier in this book, I mentioned how Dr. Price was aided by a number of leading physicians of the day. Dr. Fischer credits not only all those who worked with Dr. Price but the role of all key medical men who contributed to the basic knowledge of how infections initially originating from mild mannered, normal bacteria flora found in the mouth could become disease causing, lethal entities.

Dr. Fischer in presenting the problems had this to say:

> *"What has happened to the streptococcus we used to know that permits it to play such new and varied roles? Because of changes in its environment, the organism has been found capable of changing its qualities. Instead of the one streptococcus of classic type, there is a whole family today. Though born of a common father, as Rosenow established, the sons are possessed of unequal and different endowments. Thus all kinds are known from those that originally were not harmful in their behavior to those that become virulent and dangerous."*

During the first years of this century, it was not thought possible for organisms responsible for a specific disease to change their size, shape, virulence and staining characteristics. One of the first to discover this variability trait of certain types of bacteria was William B. Wherry, who in 1904 discovered the changeability of bacteria involved in the disease cholera.

Sometime later Dr. E.C. Rosenow reinforced Dr. Wherry's generalizations with studies of pneumococci and streptococci, finding that although they were not originally virulent, when introduced into animals they became very poisonous. He also found that when he isolated streptococcus bacteria from an infected human appendix and injected the bacteria into an animal, 80 percent developed appendicitis. In addition, he learned he could transfer bacteria in this manner from the gall bladder and that cholesystitis would occur, and that myositis (muscle inflammation) and neuritis could electively be transferred in a high percentage of cases. This work was reported in various medical journals in 1910, and in *Lancet*, the leading British medical publication, in 1914.

It was Dr. Frank Billings who first isolated bacteria from a tonsil and transferred them to an animal, causing the development of rheumatism. It was the same Billings who gave this process the name *focal infection*. Dr. Rosenow was Dr. Billings' foremost co-worker and contributed by far the greatest variety and mass of research.

We generally think of metastasis in regards to cancer. Rosenow showed how microorganisms could metastasize from a tonsil or a tooth and repeat the disease cycle in animals, just as cancer viruses travel from one organ to another.

Dr. Fischer added the following:

> *"Parlor pinks still exist who doubt the whole proposition, who believe that it cannot be so, that something else lies at the bottom of it all. For their benefit, various types of peripheral disease are now listed that have been proved to be of infectious origin and to be reproducible in exact clinical form in experimental animals by the simple process of the injection of the causative agent intravenously. The names of Billings and of Rosenow come first in this historic recital but admirable extension of the doctrine was made by some other Chicagoans — Ludvig Hektoen (the father of many children), D.J. Davis, Edwin R. LeCount, Leila Jackson, Ernest E. Irons, Rollin T. Woodyatt, George and Gladys Dick. To these may be added the names of some of Chicago's expatriates; and of some wise men who from afar observed a light — N.W. Jones, Russell L. Haden, Hermon C. Bumpus Jr., Henry A.*

Cotton, Bernard Langdon Wyatt, and Weston Price. Their combined labors made certain a new principle in clinical pathology and established a microbic origin for diseases that earlier had been attributed to evil inheritance, to the dank of draughts, high protein intakes and altitude, to the consequences of work, worry and whiskey. It is true that some of the apostles have tried to wipe the oil of their anointment from their brows but, in major portion, it has stuck."

You will note that Dr. Weston Price's name is listed among these noted physicians. Should you have been under the impression that studies of the focal infection theory were all of his doing, you can now place the whole entity in its proper perspective. Dr. Price, to my knowledge was the only dentist researching this information for the dental profession. There were others, however, who supported his endeavors.

Dr. Fischer also investigated the various organ and tissue diseases caused by focal infections quite thoroughly. Most of those he mentions were also discovered and reported by Weston Price. A brief review of the work of others involved in this research should broaden your appreciation of the depth and scope of the large number of investigations that took place so long ago.

Regarding the various heart disease problems, *endocarditis*, *pericarditis* and *myocarditis*, Drs. Billings and Rosenow were able to isolate and identify different kinds of diplococci and streptococci that were responsible for causing these heart infections. Even though heart valves had not been previously injured, he found rabbits did develop endocarditis of the heart valves after an intravenous injection of microorganisms.

These remarkable experimental findings and conclusions were confirmed by studies of doctors Drs. M.E. Winternitz, R.M. Thomas, and P.M LeCompte. It was said that such foci are reminiscent of early stage rheumatic heart muscle inflammation which is the pathologic background for the slowly progressive "chronic" heart disease that kills so many humans after age 40 but whose cause is unknown.

Then came Drs. N.W. Jones and S.J. Newsome reporting in the *Archives of Pathology* in 1932 about drilling into the pulp chambers of dogs' teeth and implanting streptococci bacteria and the usual type of fillings in those chambers. These dogs lived for months and some of them for years. However, when they were killed and autopsies run, vegetative lesions of the heart valves were found and numbers of patches of heart muscle degeneration had occurred. In other words, Jones and Newsome were able to produce experimentally progressive chronic "heart disease."

Then a year later, in 1933, Dr. Billings published his findings concerning patients who had chronic rheumatoid arthritis and had become severe invalids. In 70 patients he found the disease was due to streptococcic infection of the joints and tissues about them, and that the bacteria most commonly were traced as coming from the tonsils and, secondarily, from the teeth and sinuses.

Dr. Fischer also reported on the work of doctors Drs. E.J. Poynton and A. Paine, that rheumatism was due to a specific streptococcus. Their work found little acceptance because other researchers failed in their attempts to cultivate the organisms. In every instance it was shown that these investigators failed to follow the specialized techniques necessary to reproduce the bacteria.

Then in 1947, it was Rosenow again who, in a report in the *Journal of the American Medical Association*, told how he had produced stomach and duodenal ulcers in 18 rabbits, six dogs, and a monkey by intravenous injection of strains of streptococcus bacteria that had been obtained from tonsils and from the tissues of patients having rheumatism. He concluded that:

> *"Relation between infected tonsils or gums and gastric ulcer may be due, not to the swallowing of bacteria, but to the entrance into the blood of streptococci of the proper kind to produce a local infection in the walls of the stomach."*

Then Dr. Fischer told of streptococcus that were recovered from dental infections in patients who had pyelonephritis (kidney lesions) and how this disease was transferred to rabbits; this was the work of Drs. H.D. Bumpus and J.G. Meisser and was reported originally in the *Journal of Internal Medicine*.

Dr. Russell L. Hayden subsequently confirmed these findings by producing kidney lesions in 40 percent of 416 animals from root end infections from six patients having pyelonephritis.

These investigations, by others than Dr. Price, should be sufficient for you to see the wide scope of illnesses that can arise from teeth, tonsils, and other focal infection sites. Dr. Fischer reported many more, i.e., gall bladder disease, pneumonia, bronchitis, asthma, pleuritis, both hyper and hypo thyroidism, eye infections, herpes zoster (shingles), infection of the fingernail beds, poliomyelitis, multiple sclerosis, senility, pharyngitis, gastritis, appendicitis, colitis, and dermatitis.

Toward the end of Dr. Price's Volume I of his two books, he made this statement:

"Government statistics speak of the degenerative diseases frequently as old age diseases, and it is pathetic that so many individuals are slowly dying of old age anywhere from thirty years on."

These diseases can, of course, also occur because of other degenerative processes but it would seem prudent to first rule out teeth, tonsils and other focal infection sites as the consequences of oral infections are apt to be of a severe nature.

Summary:

- A statement that I made earlier in this book, *Root Canal Cover-up Exposed! Many Illnesses Result*, is most likely causing some of my dental colleagues to bitterly resent the charge that our profession has unknowingly been responsible for the deaths of many of our patients.

- How could I make such a statement when not a single one of all my dentist friends and acquaintances has knowingly lost a patient?! We generally have been considered a safe profession to practice, certainly not one that involves fatality.

- For dentists, physicians or patients who think I am merely being a sensationalist, this chapter which reviews the book *Death and Dentistry* by Martin H. Fischer, M.D. may help put this whole subject in its true perspective.

- Dr. Fisher's book states that the microorganisms from teeth and tonsils metastasize to other organs and tissues, similar to the phenomenon that occurs in cancer and 'results in similar disagreeable circumstances.'

- Dr. Fischer, a professor of physiology, reminds us that the heart disease problems of endocarditis, pericarditis and myocarditis were found to be caused by streptococci and diplococci bacteria, and that these bacteria are also found in chronic appendicitis and bleeding ulcer cases, plus gall bladder and liver diseases. We all know of people who die of these afflictions despite antibiotics. A good many of them have immune systems that have been overtaxed for long periods of time by hidden focal infections and their toxins. Such people more readily develop pneumonia or some other affliction that eventually causes their demise.

- Dr. Fischer reported how Dr. E.C. Rosenow (not Milton Rosenau, a Price Research Institute advisor) isolated streptococcus bacteria from a human infected appendix and injected these bacteria into animals, 80 percent of which developed appendicitis. The same Dr. Rosenow reported in the *AMA Journal* how he had produced stomach and duodenal ulcers in 18 rabbits, six dogs and a monkey by inoculating these animals with bacteria from the tonsils and the tissues of patients with rheumatism.

- Dr. Rosenow stated that most doctors think ulcers in the stomach are due to the patient swallowing bacteria from infected tonsils or teeth, but he contends that their mode of spread is through the bloodstream.

- Dr. Fischer's book is full of studies similar to those I have mentioned in this chapter which confirm Price's discoveries.

- Like the investigators of this subject named in Dr. Fischer's book, other outstanding leaders in this field of research are: Frank Billings, Milton Rosenow, Ludvig Hektoen, D.J. Davis, Edwin LeCount, Leila Jackson, Ernest E. Irons, Rollin T. Woodyatt, George and Gladys Dick, N.W. Jones, Russell Haden, Herman C. Burnpus, Jr., Henry A. Cotton, Bernard Langdon Wyatt, and Weston Price.

- Each person listed above significantly contributed to setting up of a new paradigm, a new basic principle in clinical bacteriology and pathology.

- All of the charges that degenerative diseases are the result of poor inheritance; too much or too little protein, vitamins or minerals; too much beer, wine or whiskey; and the overuse of sugar, sweets and caffeine products, while partially the case, must not deter serious consideration of those 24 million root canal treatments performed last year, not to mention the billion or so that exist in mouths of people throughout America and the rest of the world.

CHAPTER 23

The Fantastic Scanning Electron Microscope
See Infection Causing Bacteria Magnified the Size of Peas!

Early in my reading of the Price root canal books, I came across the microscope picture he made showing the presence of bacteria inside dentin tubules. Until I saw that picture of Dr. Price's, never in all my schooling nor in 47 years of practice did I ever see a picture of bacteria in dentin tubules.

Inasmuch as the bacteria seen in old microscopes appeared merely as black dots that some believed were metabolic debris, it occurred to me that research pictures using modern electron scanning microscopes would show organisms and dentin tubules to better advantage. More recent graduates of dental schools are no doubt well aware of this phenomenon.

For those of you not familiar with the scanning electron microscope, it is one in which the object is examined point by point directly by an electronic beam. The image is not viewed in a scope but is formed and transmitted to a television screen. With this method, an unembedded specimen is viewed by reflected electrons and secondary electrons, thereby giving the objects being viewed an image that is three-dimensional.

In order to obtain information about the most recent work along these lines, I telephoned the librarian at the American Dental Association office in Chicago requesting articles showing electron microscope pictures of bacteria in dental tubules. My request was granted by way of a loan of two books from the A.D.A. Library. The first is one by Swedish dental researcher, Dr. Martin Brännström.

It contains magnificent color and black and white photographs of the different parts of teeth, including enamel, dentin, and pulp, and many do show the presence of bacteria in dentin tubules. You will note that in some of the pictures taken from his book, *Dentin and Pulp in Restorative Dentistry*, that the bacteria appear almost as large as marbles.

I telephoned Dr. Brännström in Stockholm and asked if he had carried out any work with teeth that had root canal fillings. He said that he had not done so nor could I find any others who had done so.

Dr. Brännström gave me permission to use the pictures that follow in this chapter. His book was published by Wolfe Publishing in England, 1982. It is one of the titles in the series, *Wolfe Medical Atlases*, which brings together possibly the world's largest systematic published collection of color photographs of medical and dental subject matter.

The following scanning electron microscope pictures are the result of magnification of between 1,000 and 15,000 times. This magnitude of enlargement will provide you with a much better understanding of the complications involved in this subject. It is very difficult to believe that these tiny hollow tubes are so small they can only be seen with the aid of a

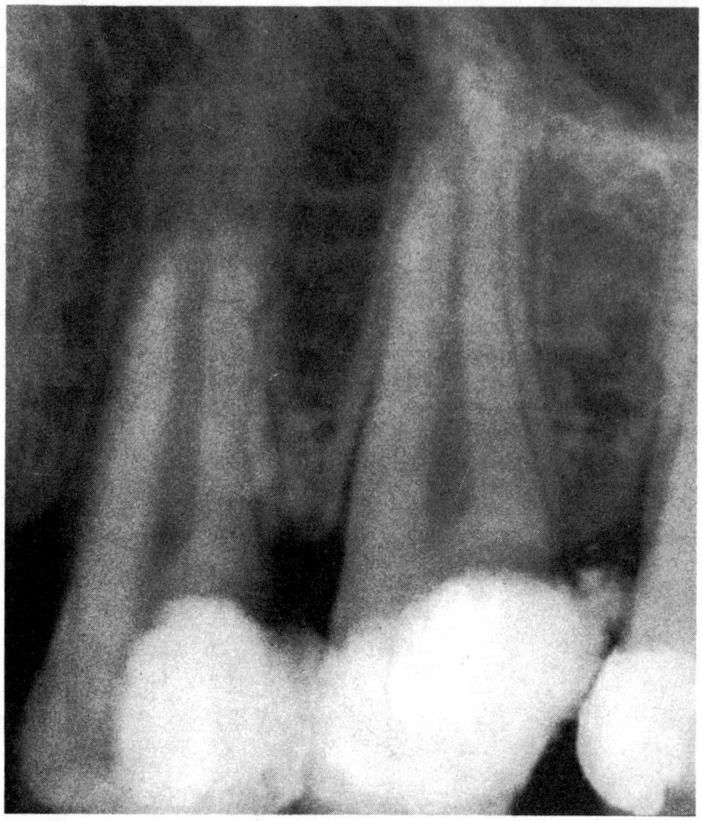

Figure 1

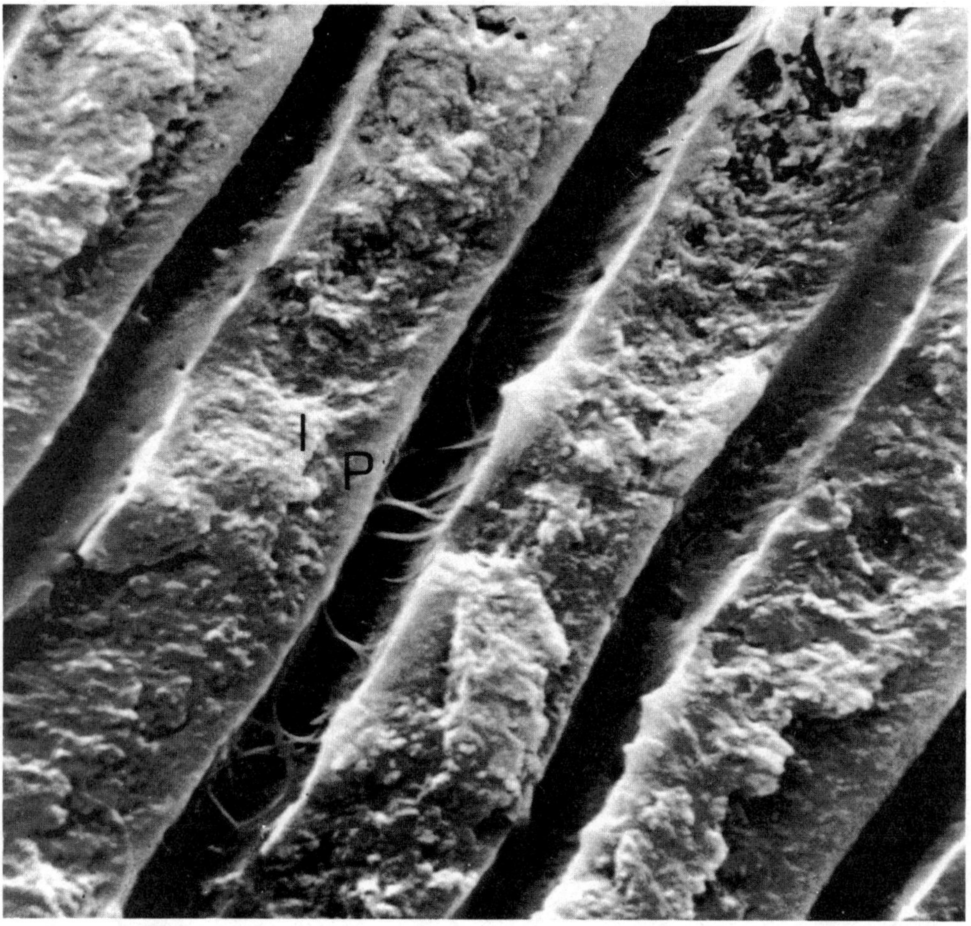

Figure 2: x 6,000

tiny hollow tubes are so small they can only be seen with the aid of a microscope. In fact they are so small that between 20,000 and 45,000 of them will fit into one square millimeter of space. A millimeter is roughly one thirty-second of an inch. Though hard to believe, that is exactly what you will be seeing greatly magnified in these pictures.

The first picture on the preceding page, Figure 1, is of two teeth whose vital pulps (nerves) have been exposed by very deep seated tooth decay. Just how the bacteria involved in such cavities in teeth can be responsible for a vast number of degenerative diseases has been the main subject of this book. The viewing of these scanning electron microscope pictures will enable you to see how easy it is for microorganisms to reside in the tubules but the mystery of how they mutate and become so virulent still escapes us.

The second picture on the preceding page, Figure 2, magnified 6,000 times, shows a longitudinal view of three dentin tubules and part of a fourth. The section of tooth involved is just 1.2 millimeters into the dentin from its border with the pulp. It should be noted that the wall or collar of the dentin tubule is quite hard and dense. It is called peritubular dentin, "P." The structure that connects and holds the tubules in place is called the intertubular dentin, "I."

The picture below shows dentin tubules cut in cross section. The one on the left, Figure 3, was magnified 1120 times; the one on the right, Figure 4, 5000 times. The larger one was treated with citric acid for one minute. This removes the fibrils between the tubules, making the tubules more visible.

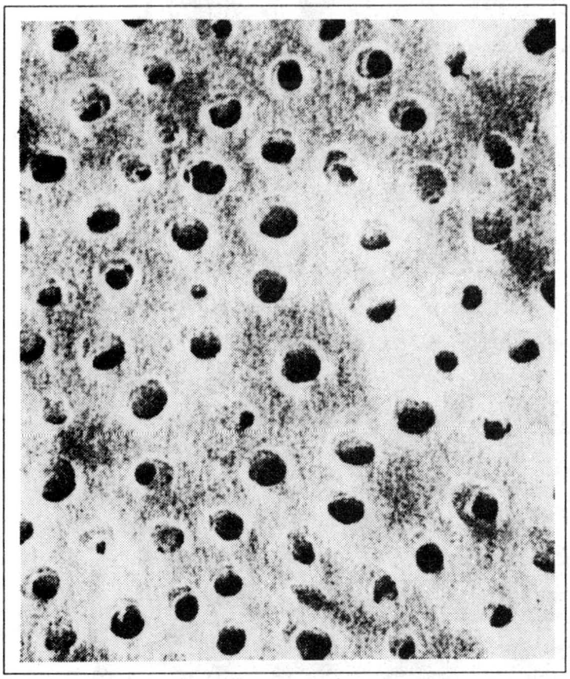

Figure 3: x 1,120

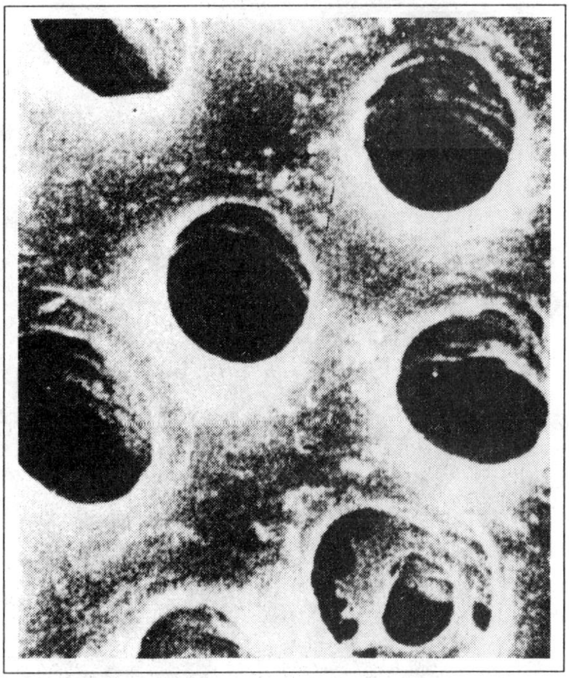

Figure 4: x 5,000

The structure between the tubules is a matrix consisting of bundles of collagen fibrils that run at right angles to the tubules. The fibrils contain mineral crystals that align themselves with the highly mineralized matrix. It is these minerals that are partially responsible for the hardness of teeth and bring attention once again to the importance of diet to the health of teeth. You will recall that in an earlier chapter I mentioned how dentin tubules contain a fluid and that this fluid moves from the pulp in the inside of the tooth outwardly, carrying nutrients that nourish our teeth.

In the next interesting picture, Figure 5, just the first superficial layer of dentin substance was dissolved away by the action of citric acid. It will be noted that the tubules seem wider and that the fibril structure of the intertubular dentin that helps hold the tubules to one another are more clearly visible. Because of our interest in the microorganisms in teeth, of even greater interest are the clusters of bacteria that are readily visible and the aperture opening of the tubules. Two good examples are labeled "B" in the center of the picture.

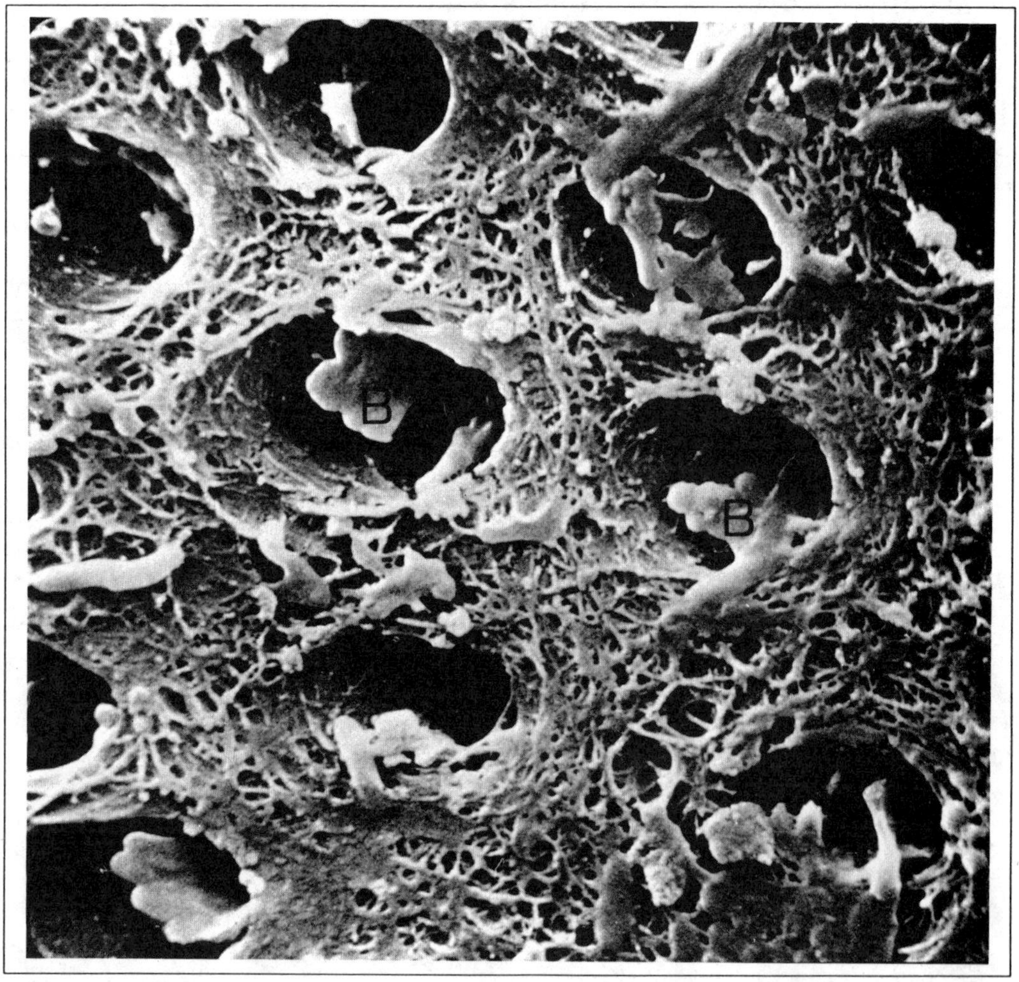

Figure 5: x 5,500

A crack that was created in the extracted tooth produced a most informative picture as is seen in the scanning electron microscope view, Figure 6, shown below. Not only are the dentin tubules seen in cross section but they can be observed longitudinally as well. Close observation discloses the tubules to be somewhat tunnel shaped.

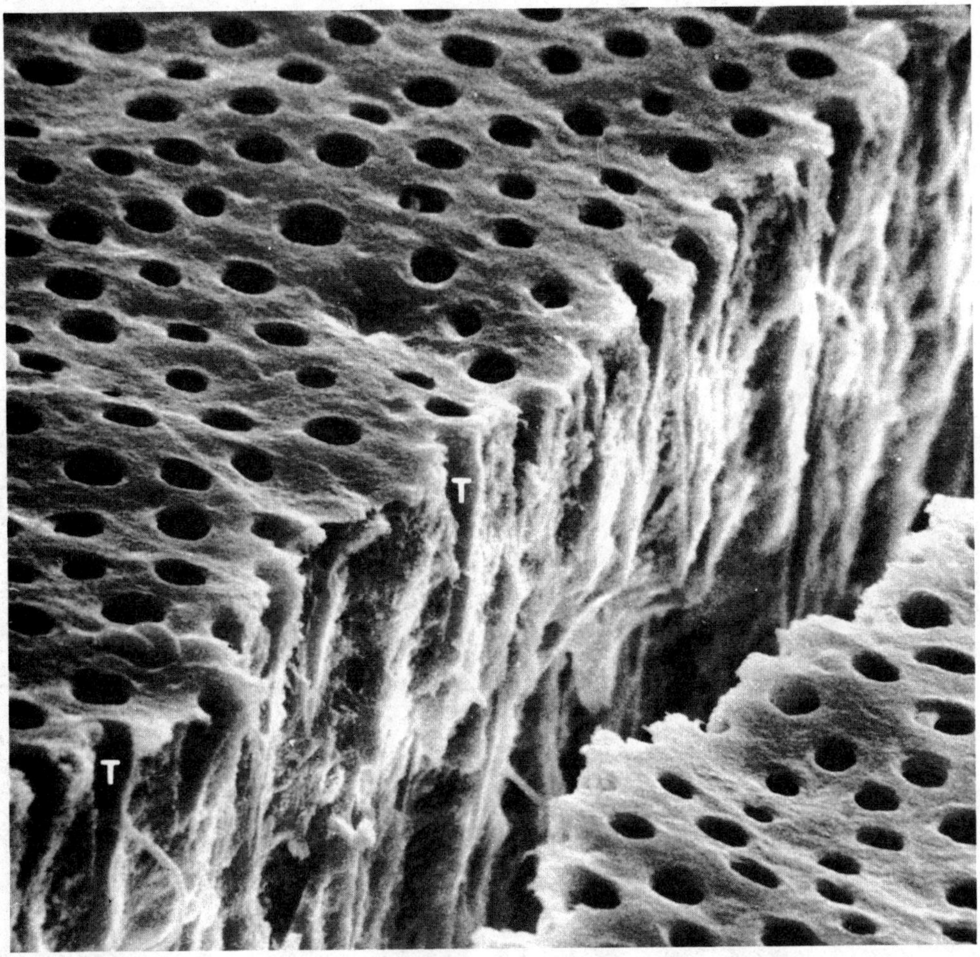

Figure 6: x 1,210

The tooth in the lower picture had beginning decay that seemed to be limited to the enamel fissure in the crown. The brown color of decayed tooth structure was evident although the caries had not progressed out of the enamel into the dentin. A yellow staining of the first dentin tubules was evident. The investigators also found that the dentin between the tubules was finely granulated and the fibril structure was no longer visible. One tubule in the picture has lost its pertubular wall or collar, "T." This section of the tooth is only one millimeter in from the enamel junction into the dentin but a beginning invasion of numerous, multiplying cocci bacteria can readily be observed. This means that shallow tooth decay is much deeper into the tooth than we dentists have ever imagined. The magnification in this study, Figure 7, on the left was 6,500 times. Figure 8, on the right, was magnified 12,500 times.

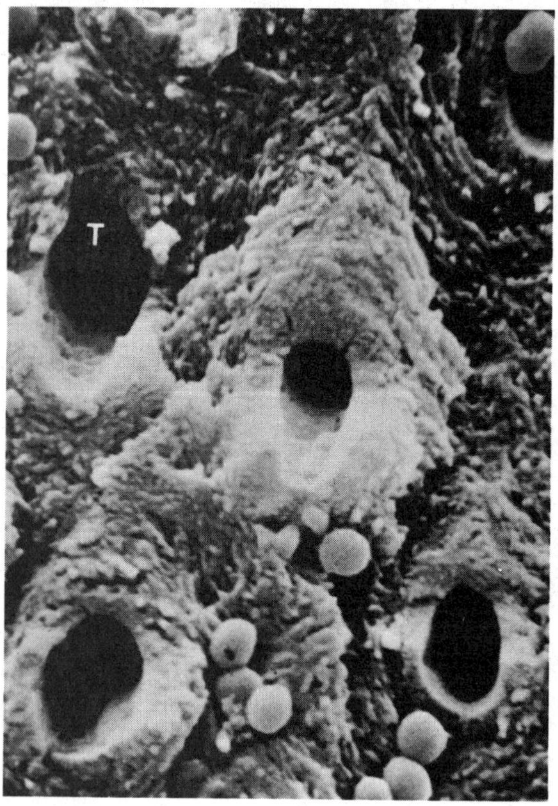

Figure 7: x 6,500

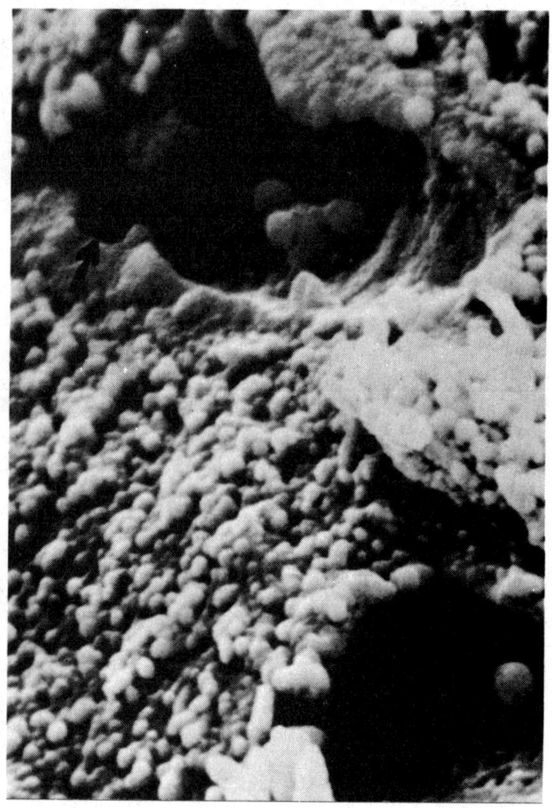

Figure 8.: x 12,500

The very first sign of the presence of tooth decay is a white chaulky area on the surface of the enamel before any cavitation takes place. The enamel's structure, unlike that of the dentin, is composed of enamel rods or prisms. The picture on the left, Figure 9, shows the enamel rods and bacteria attacking the structure in-between the enamel rods. The picture on the right Figure 10, is taken at a slightly advanced stage, showing the beginning destruction of an enamel rod, many round cocci, and rod shaped bacilli present in-between the prisms.

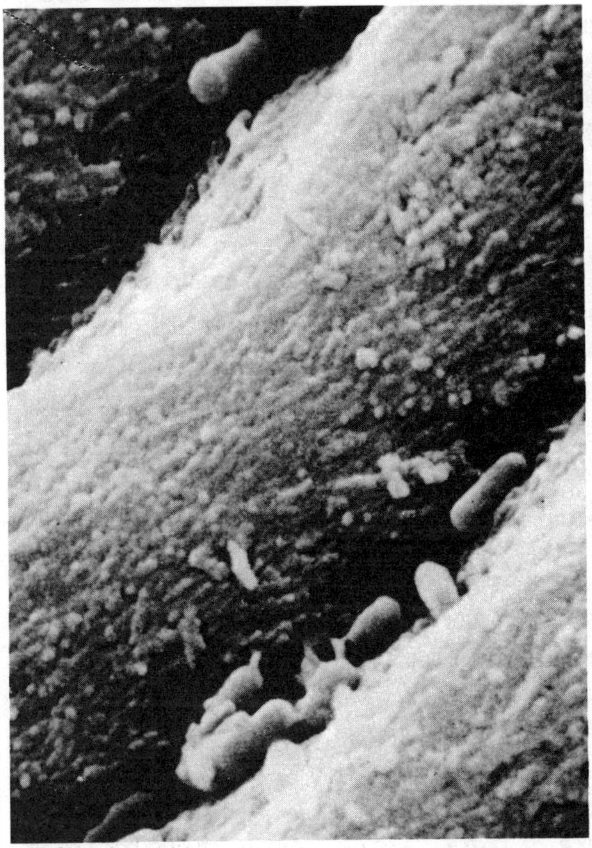

Figure 9: x 8,000

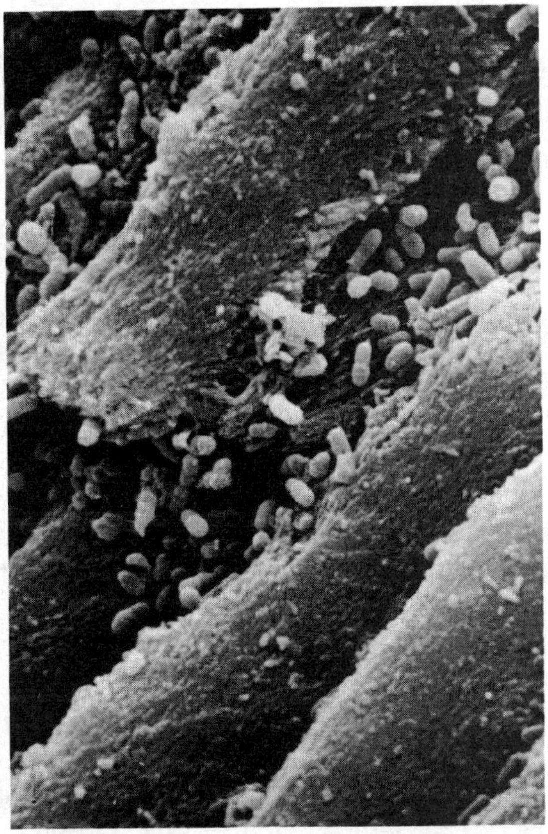

Figure 10: x 4,000

The second book the American Dental Association Library made available to me was a record of papers submitted at a symposium held at the University of Dundee, Scotland in 1967. Some 30 scientists who were leaders of their institutions in the fields of preventive dentistry, anatomy, pathology, cytochemistry, oral biology, morphology, and endocrinology presented electron microscope research papers that were published in book form under the title *Dentin and the Pulp*.

However, in reading the reports of the 30 leading research scientists presented in this book, none were related to the work Dr. Price had conducted regarding organisms he found in root canal filled teeth.

The information presented in the symposium book mainly concerns the conduction of pain in teeth; how the decay process advances; what happens inside of teeth when they are prepared for fillings and crowns; what happens under fillings; what factors are involved when teeth are sensitive from erosion, abrasion, fractures, and injuries; and a host of other data — all of which broadens our knowledge regarding teeth.

A major part of all the different presentations at this symposium concerned the fluid movement inside dentin tubules and causative factors that detrimentally influence reactions that take place in the pulp tissue. Though research has been going on in this field since Dr. Fish first reported fluid movement in dentin tubules in 1927, it is mainly since the 60s that the majority of contributions have been made.

Professor I.R.H. Kramer of London, in his concluding summary of the seminar, stated that many of the most important contributions in this field have come from Dr. Brännström and his colleagues, and that their work has contributed greatly to understanding how the living pulp tissue inside of teeth responds to the variety of operation procedures of dentists and the materials and drugs they use.

In researching literature for data that might show support for the Price revelations of so long ago, I also came across an article by L.M. Silverstone and M.J. Hicks that appeared in *Gerodontics* in 1985:1:185-193 under the title, "The Structure and Ultra Structure of the Carious Lesion in Human Dentin."

Their electron microscope pictures, though quite similar to those of Dr. Brännström, show a somewhat different appearance so I am presenting these pictures taken by two investigators from another country, Denmark.

The upper picture, Figure 11, on the next page is taken through a fracture area.

The lower picture, Figure 12, is taken under higher magnification and indicates the tubules to be about 2.5 microns in diameter. They are surrounded by highly mineralized collars and the matrix between the tubules consists of bundles of collagen fibrils that run at right angles to the tubules. Mineral crystals that give strength to the dentin can also be seen among the fibrils. The fracture area through the tubules differs from that of the highly mineralized matrix.

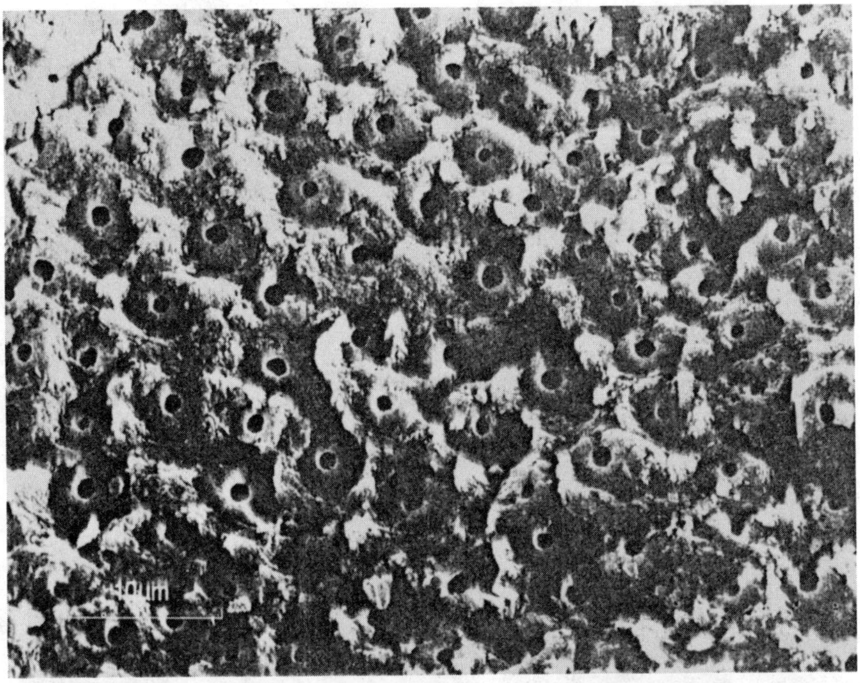

Figure 11

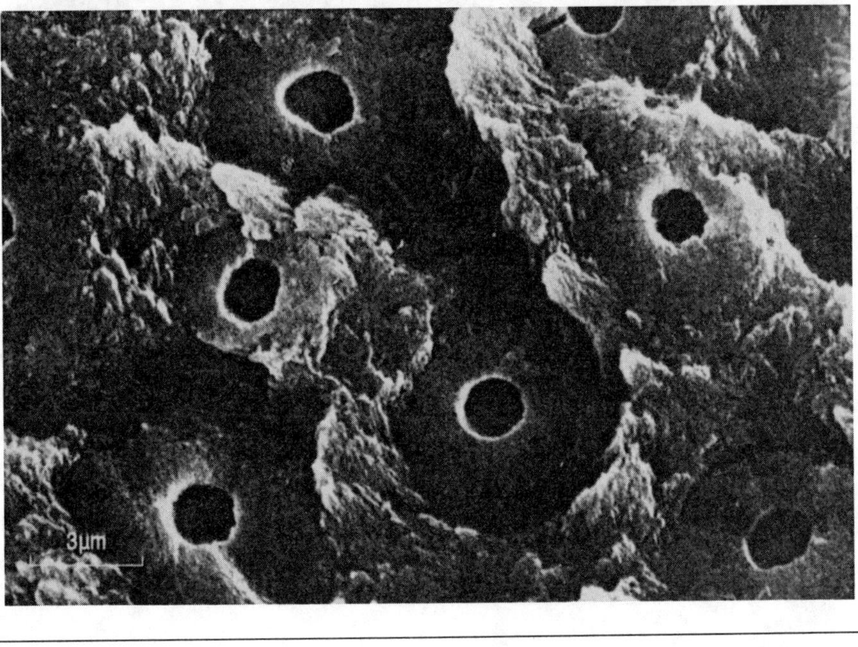

Figure 12

This next picture, Figure 13, was made after the peritubular matrix and the tubular contents were removed to explore the character of the dentin. The dentin was treated with phosphoric acid, which Silverstone and Hicks used instead of the citric acid employed by Dr. Brännström for this purpose. The collagenous dentin between the tubules can be seen as a dense matrix.

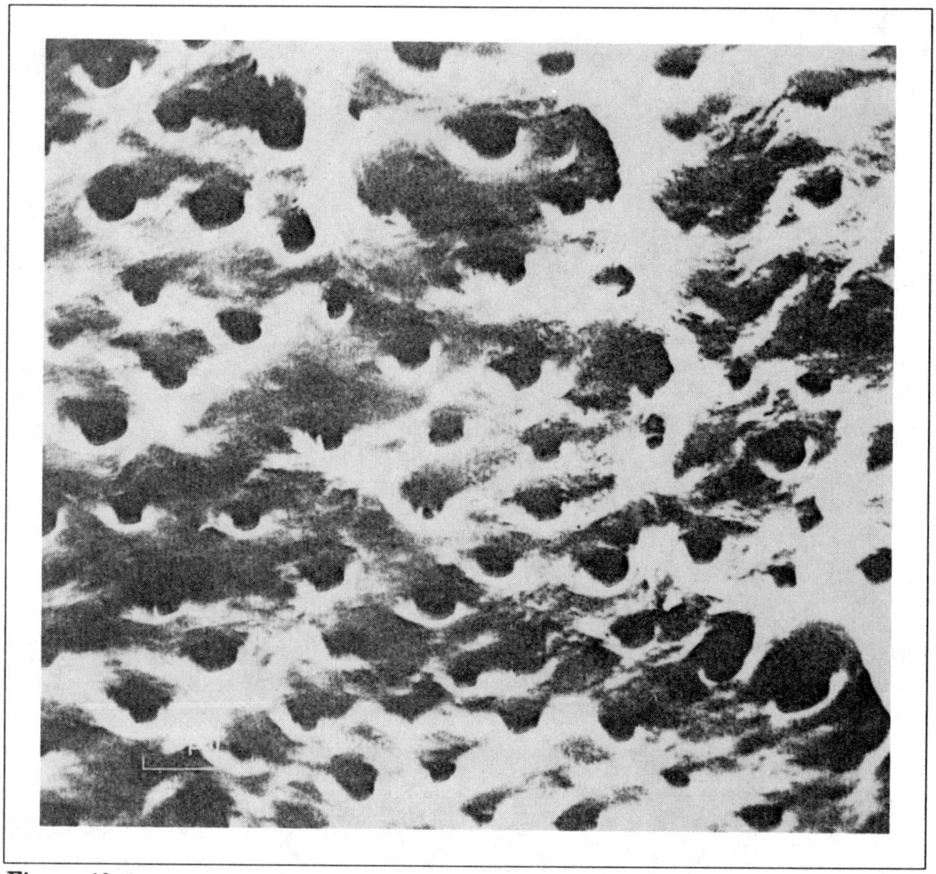

Figure 13

Permission to reproduce these last three pictures was kindly permitted by the publishers of the Dr. L.M. Silverstone and Dr. M.J. Hicks *Gerodontics* article in 1985, namely Munksgard Publishing Ltd. of Copenhagen, Denmark, 25/9/92.

I was fortunate to be able to reproduce the prior scanning electron microscope pictures in this chapter and some of the accompanying data due to the courtesy and permission of the author, Dr. Brännström of Stockholm, Sweden and the publishers of his book, *Dentin and the Pulp in Restorative Dentistry*, Wolfe Publishing, Mosby Year Book Europe, Ltd., Brookhouse, 2-16 Torrington Place, London, WC1E 7LT, England.

Summary:

- Of particular interest in my investigation of scanning electron microscope pictures, other than the revealing magnified size of the bacteria, was finding that scientists using these instruments have not investigated bacteria in dentin tubules of root canal filled teeth.
- This has been a disappointment as pictures of bacteria inside dentin tubules would no doubt broaden our understanding of how these organisms adjust and adapt to such unfavorable conditions, and how their destructive toxins are produced.
- This is not to detract from the outstanding results of these microscopic investigations, as their contributions to our understanding of what goes on in teeth are advancing dentistry by fantastic leaps and bounds.
- Dr. Brännström's work in Stockholm proved particularly impressive.
- It is hard to believe that the dentin tubules that make up the majority of the hard substance of teeth are made up of tiny hollow tubes so small that 30,000 of them occupy a space of one square millimeter — a little less than a 32nd of an inch.
- It is even harder to believe that the two holes on Figure 8, having a diameter of an inch and a half, are a magnified cross section of a dentin tubule — and the pea size substances floating in the tubules are bacteria.
- Figures 9 and 10 show what the rods that make up enamel look like when magnified and how bacteria attack between the rods at the beginning moments of the tooth decay process.
- Figure 6 is an exceptionally beautiful picture of a crack through dentin that shows the dentin tubules not only in cross section (the round holes) but also their longitudinal course and that they are tapered or funnel shaped.
- The other pictures are various views at different magnitudes.

CHAPTER 24

Chronic Infected Holes Left in Jaw Bones After Tooth Extraction (Neuralgia-inducing Cavitational Osteonecrosis)

Extraction Protocol

If those chapter titles and subtitles are not formidable enough, let me add: *"Just pulling the tooth is not enough when tooth removal proves necessary."*

In an earlier chapter, I mentioned that Price found bacteria in the tissues and bone just adjacent to the tooth's root when he biopsied a section from this area and looked at it under a microscope. He felt the bacteria contained therein were coming from the root filled tooth.

During the early 1950s it was noted by some European physicians and dentists that the sockets of numbers of old tooth extraction sites had not filled in completely, thereby leaving thin holes in the bones of the jaw — and even larger areas at times.

These cavitations result when the periodontal ligament, the tough fibrous tissue that holds the root of a tooth to its bony socket, does not break down and disappear during the healing process. Thus, as the socket fills in with new bone, this thin strip of fibrous tissue leaves a narrow space that contains whatever bacteria and toxins that have traveled there from the infected tooth.

In addition, lymphocytes (white blood cells formed in lymph tissues) are found in the areas of the periodontal ligament and its adjoining jaw bone. The white blood cells are present to control the disease activity that now remains to plague the patient's immune system.

Microscopic biopsies show that very few bacteria are present in these cavitation areas, but scavenger cells (macrophages) that ingest foreign materials are numerous. Their function isn't completely clear as yet, but they aren't nearly as efficient as polymorphonuclear leucocytes, the tongue twister name for a specialized type of white blood cell important in removing bacteria and toxic substances.

Incidentally, this phenomenon of the infections of teeth invading the wall of the tooth socket was also recognized and written about by Martin Fischer, M.D. in his book discussed in Chapter 23.

This means that in order to prevent the formation of these areas of infection when infected teeth are extracted, it would be prudent for the dentist to remove the periodontal ligament and one millimeter of the bony socket.

Dentists are accustomed to always curette away the soft infected tissue granulomas and cysts at the end of the roots of infected teeth. However, the thought of removing, at the same time, one millimeter of the entire bony socket will probably seem farfetched and ridiculous. However, preventing these cavitation areas from forming is a necessary disease prevention procedure. What is more, it is quite simple, quick, and painless.

Though little about this subject is known to the average dentist and physician, it is beginning to receive the attention of health care professionals as one of the most neglected and ignored areas related to the incidence of degenerative, chronic disease. That dearth of knowledge is now being satisfied by the appearance of numbers of articles and research reports. In California during February 1993, an informative three day seminar on this subject was presented by an outstanding faculty of physicians, dentists and Ph.D.'s from various parts of the world. The impeccable scholastic backgrounds of the speakers advanced materially the understanding of this little known subject.

Over the years dentists have had visits from a relatively small number of patients who complain of obscure pains in the mouth, face and jaws. These are generally chronic, long-term events that vary from mild to very severe as in the case of trigeminal neuralgia.

Dr. J.E. Bouquot et al. in an article in the *Journal of Oral Surgery, Oral Medicine and Oral Pathology* reported in March of 1992 some 1995 cases of neuralgia osteonecrosis. The individual totals were published for each of the various cases from 1976 through 1991.

Most of these diseased areas are not easy to distinguish on x-ray films. However, when they are surgically explored, there is no question that the tissue removed is abnormal. It has been described as "gritty," "like sawdust," "a hollow cavity," "has small clips or flakes of dead bone," "dry but some tend to bleed."

Dr. Bouquot and his group reported on 103 cases in 1991 of which 34 were trigeminal neuralgia patients. They found by surgically eliminating these areas in the jaws that 73 percent had total relief and 16 percent moderate relief, but that the patients were satisfied with their program. When you consider that most people suffering this affliction have been going from dentist to dentist and physician to physician for many years trying to solve their pain problem, you can see why the recognition of this disease entity is an important one.

Since becoming aware of this problem about a year ago, I have had the chance to advise one woman about this procedure. She suffered almost daily for over three years and spent great sums on ineffective treatments, antibiotics and other drugs. She is now one happy person.

Like many newly discovered illnesses, it is difficult to know what to call them. Each investigator seems to delight in presenting ideas for a name. At first these cavitation areas were just called "holes in the bone." Then they became "alveolar cavitation pathosis," and that was followed by "alveolar

0steo pathosis." Perhaps now "neuralgia-inducing cavitational osteo necrosis" (NICO) will stick. I mention all these names only so those who suffer this illness will be able to identify it when it is described by name.

Most reports about these cases in dental literature do not mention the relationship of how tooth infections can involve the periodontal membrane, the tough fibrous tissue that holds the tooth to the bony socket, and how infection therein can become trapped in the jaw.

Avoiding this problem requires a relatively simple procedure be undertaken immediately after infected teeth are removed. Inasmuch as evidence points to the accumulation of bacteria and their toxins in the periodontal membrane and the first millimeter of the bony socket, these tissues must be removed to prevent the possibility of the formation of cavitations and neuralgic complications.

The following protocol when followed is not only preventive of future trouble but promotes a better recovery from any degenerative process that is due to root canal infection.

PROTOCOL for REMOVAL of a ROOT FILLED TOOTH

For those dentists and oral surgeons who want to truly restore the health of patients whose root canal filled teeth are to be removed, the following protocol is strongly suggested. This is not the only way this procedure can be carried out but it is one that has been used very successfully since 1990.

After the tooth has been removed, slow-speed drilling with number 8 round burr is used to remove one millimeter of the entire bony socket, including the apex area.

The purpose of the procedure is to remove the periodontal ligament and the first millimeter of bone as they are usually infected with toxins that are produced by streptococcus bacteria living in the dentin tubules. The periodontal ligament is always infected, and most of the time the bone will also be infected.

While this procedure is being done, irrigate the socket with sterile saline via a Monoject 412, 12cc syringe. This has a curved plastic tip and is very handy in carrying out the procedure. Two or three syringes of solution may be needed, but they are much easier to use than one large 50cc syringe. The purpose of the flushing action is to remove the contaminated bone as it is cut.

In cutting the bone, not only are the toxins removed, but the bone is "perturbed." This perturbation of the bone stimulates a change from osteocytes to osteoblasts. The blast cells are the ones that generate new bone formation.

After the socket has been cut, it should be filled with a *non-vasoconstrictor* anesthetic. Allow the liquid local anesthetic to set for about thirty (30) seconds.

Next, suction should be applied gently to the socket area so that the majority of the anesthetic is removed, but there is still a substantial coating of the anesthetic over the bony interior. This further perturbs the bone cells to encourage osteoblastic action and bone healing.

The use of PZI (protamine zinc insulin suspension USP) is recommended for those people who are familiar with its usages; three units is adequate.

It is believed that the use of antibiotics may convert the osteoblasts back into osteocytes, leaving a cap of bone over the socket area; but the internal portion may not heal and years later may be found to be an empty socket lined by the deleterious effects of the autoimmune process.

The simple procedures provided in this protocol may be copied by readers or by dentists, physicians, or other health practitioners in order to assure that patients having infected teeth removed will also have all adjoining infected tissue removed, thereby providing for full return to health.

Incidentally, when this protocol is followed, the tooth socket heals much more rapidly, with less bleeding and pain.

Summary:

- Although Price, using biopsies of the bone next to the root of an infected tooth found that the bone contained bacteria, it was felt at that time that these areas healed satisfactorily when the infected tooth was extracted.

- Dentists have always advocated curetting away or surgically removing granulomas and cysts in tooth sockets after extractions but it is only in recent years that the problem of cavitations has been recognized. However, Dr. Fischer in his book, *Death and Dentistry*, did mention cavitations in the 1940s and that they were involved in the infection problem.

- Cavitations are areas that arise when the periodontal ligament that holds the tooth to its bony socket and that first millimeter of infected bone fails to be destroyed by the healing process after tooth extraction.

- Sometimesa cavitation shows up on x-ray pictures as a thin space in the bone — in other words, a hole. Other times, nothing is seen on x-rays, but when the areas are entered surgically, the bone has a gritty, sawdust-like consistency and the area contains some small chip of dead bone.

- Microscopic studies of the tissues in these areas show very few bacteria but macrophages are present. Macrophages do not seem to be as efficient in clearing away infection materials and their toxins as do white blood cells.

- What has been discovered is that these areas — now called *cavitational osteopathosis* (ACOs) and more recently, *neuralgia inducing cavitational osteonecrosis* (NICO) — are capable of producing long-term neurologic pain and, in some cases, a continuation of degenerative disease problems.

- When dentists surgically clean out these areas, the long-term symptoms disappear.

- Don't be surprised if your dentist knows very little about cavitation areas. He or she can obtain articles about scientific studies on the subject from the American Dental Association Library Service.

- An important part of this chapter is the detailing of the protocol that should be followed after a tooth that has a root canal filling is extracted. This is usually a simple procedure. It ensures all infected material in the tooth socket is removed, thereby preventing later cavitation areas from occurring.

- This protocol can be copied from the book and given to your dentist so he or she can prevent the retention of any infected material in your tooth socket. Better yet, he or she can be given a copy of this book.

CHAPTER 25

Conclusions

There have been times in man's research for the control of disease when great discoveries have become mired in such negative controversy that their benefits to mankind have been lost for long periods of time. A typical example has been the conflict that took place over the focal infection theory during the first two decades of this century.

The important, significant research about this subject that was conducted by some of this country's leading physicians and by research dental specialist Dr. Weston Price is finally being brought to light by the publication of this book.

In exposing the destructive focal infection side effects arising in teeth and tonsils, it is my fervent hope that you will be awakened to the benefits and improvements that can occur to your personal health and to that of your family.

It is certainly unfortunate that all of these important discoveries were forced underground and lost to the world as it is quite likely that solutions to the effective sterilization of the bacteria that invade dentin tubules would by now have been determined.

Understanding the focal infection theory is not too difficult. It contends that an infection somewhere in the body can be transported from its original location and reappear in another organ or tissue. At first it seems unbelievable that 90 percent of such infections start in teeth and tonsils.

The complexities involved in understanding tooth infections concern the nature of dentin tubules and how these harmless bacteria that reside in our mouths can become so virulent as to cause serious and even fatal degenerative disease conditions.

Through modern electron microscope pictures we have been given the ability to see these extremely tiny dentin tubules that make up most of our tooth structure and the bacteria that become trapped therein.

The greatest difficulty most have is in accepting the polymorphic characteristics of these particular groups of bacteria. Their ability to change, adapt, mutate, become smaller and more virulent, and for their toxins to become more toxic, does challenge our belief systems. But we have seen the pictures of hearts, kidneys, eyes, sex organs, and other tissues of rabbits after teeth containing bacteria have been imbedded under their skins and the wide divergence of degenerative diseases that have resulted.

In thousands of experiments, the tissues most often infected were those of the heart. In Price's two volume report of his research, heart conditions appear more often than all the other degenerative diseases combined.

Heart disease is our nation's number one killer, causing close to a million deaths a year. Reducing that figure would be a significant accomplishment.

Diseases of the heart are formidable. One fifth of heart disease victims die before the age of 65. Even worse, five percent die before 45 years of age.

In view of the important role that Price and others found of streptococcus and other oral bacteria in the cause of heart disease, and considering that the number of deaths from this illness have increased since Price's time from 10 percent to more than half of all deaths currently, the dental profession must, in good conscience, reassess its involvement and responsibilities regarding the appalling number of fatalities annually of this disorder.

The cost of heart surgeries in the U.S. in 1987 was $7,560,000 and the total cost of medical care of heart patients in that year amounted to 41 billion dollars. You can see why the government might look favorably upon disclosures that could materially reduce these figures.

Though infections of hearts predominated, there was hardly any degenerative disease that didn't result from tooth infections. But that's not all. Each of the illnesses that occurred were often a reflection of body chemistry changes also taking place due to the infection. Many of these changes noted by Dr. Price are of significance. I will reiterate some of his important disclosures.

- Dental focal infections, in many instances, lower the ionic calcium of the blood.

- If blood is withdrawn from a patient who is suffering from one of a number of degenerative diseases, and an infected tooth from that patient is extracted and placed in a vessel containing their own blood serum, the ionic calcium in that serum is markedly lowered.

- The blood of individuals suffering from degenerative lesions had lowered levels of ionic calcium, and the total combined calcium of these patients was extremely low. However, the ill health conditions usually progressively disappeared after a dental infection was removed.

- When an infected tooth of a patient was placed under the skin of a rabbit, the animal experienced a similar reduced ionic calcium of its blood and malfunctions of the glands of internal secretion were produced.

- When organisms originating from infected teeth were grown in culture and injected into animals, they produced changes in the animal's blood, including a reduction in ionic calcium.

- Dental infections reduced the body's normal alkaline reserve in the blood of both patients and animals; that is, they produced acidosis.

- In some cases it was found that a patient's blood sugar content would return to normal after the removal of infected teeth, and the blood sugar of animals was found to increase when injected with a culture from such teeth.

- The presence of dental infections increases the uric acid of the blood.

- When patients have a liberal loss of bone from dental infections, they will generally have a high ionic calcium level in the blood. Conversely, those with a tendency towards the development and deposition of calcium, such as in condensing osteitis and osteoarthritis cases, tend to have low ionic calcium of the blood.

- People who have a marked tendency to develop tooth decay (dental caries) have, at that time, an ionic calcium level that is below normal. Conversely, individuals with complete freedom from caries almost always have an ionic calcium level of the blood that is at or above normal.

- Persons who normally have a persistent low ionic calcium of the blood tend to have denser bones and some difficulty in becoming anesthetized; individuals with a normally high ionic calcium of the blood tend to have bones that are looser knit and less dense and they readily respond to local anesthetics.

- Low ionic calcium individuals tend to heal slowly and have a marked tendency to develop secondary infections of sockets following extraction; whereas individuals with high ionic calcium almost invariably experience rapid repair and seldom develop secondary infections.

- Those who experience the so-called "dry socket" and suffer its painful course are almost always those who, at the time, have a low ionic calcium level of the blood.

- People with low ionic calcium and with condensing osteitis tend, after tooth extractions, to have spicules of bone work loose from the socket, while individuals with high ionic calcium levels rarely develop this problem.

- Individuals with high ionic calcium of the blood tend, quite regularly, to develop periodontal disease; whereas patients with low ionic calcium do not tend toward the development of gum diseases.

- When infected teeth are placed under the skin of rabbits, there is almost always a reduction of the ionic calcium of the blood, and as death approaches ionic calcium levels decrease progressively; death generally occurs when the calcium gets to a low of 6 or 7 milligrams.

- Life in every form is dependent on free ionic calcium.

Some of my dentist friends and others who are aware that I am writing this book have expressed concern over the criticism I may receive in exposing this root canal information cover-up to the public. I anticipate some very tough technical questions and, for some, I may not have answers. However, considering that 17,390,000 root canals were performed in 1977 and that the number increased to 24,000,000 last year, I thoroughly believe that the focal infection threat from these teeth is one the public will want to know about.

If I were not willing to face the criticism, I am would not have dared to write this book for the public. It will also be read by professionals, but had I directed it toward the doctors of medicine and dentistry, I am afraid that the general public would not hear of the problems for many years to come. The information would be buried again while Price's research was repeated. There are millions of people affected by these infections, some seriously, and they have a right to personally consider their options — *now*.

All of this can certainly result in some disruption of the everyday practices of both dentists and physicians. While I am concerned about upsetting the status quo, I have come around to believing every health professional who becomes fully acquainted with the evidence by their dedication to humanity, see that the benefits of this research reaches their patients.

Luc De Schepper, M.D., Ph.D., CA, author of the book *Peak Immunity*, brings the matter into proper perspective by pointing out that it is no longer a secret that disorders that disrupt the immune system have reached epidemic proportions in this country and the world.

While the disclosures of the Dr. Price research will be particularly difficult for the members of the American Association of Endodontists, I came away from their 50th Anniversary meeting feeling confident that they will set in motion a wide variety of endeavors to solve the problems of controlling bacteria that infect dentin tubules.

The public should be aware that last year, when the AAE members were asked what would be the three key issues facing them in the next three years, 40 percent stated infection control would be their biggest concern. I am sure some were thinking of this in terms of the infections of teeth, but there is no doubt that the biggest worry is control of the AIDS virus.

In the same survey, 45 percent felt the use of lasers would be a positive factor in the treatment of root canals. I hope that techniques will be forthcoming that will solve dentin tubule sterilization problems, and the use of lasers is a possibility.

Saving teeth is such an important issue for the public and endodontists that I am sure we will continue to respect the wisdom in a statement made by my professor, Dr. Edgar Coolidge, that "Dentists can't learn how to save teeth by taking them out."

Throughout this book I have presented data that repeatedly underlines the genius of Weston Price and his activities. The thoroughness with which his projects were performed was exemplary. The extensive technical data in his two books is overwhelming. Following is a short review of their contents.

Book I contains: 703 pages, including 262 illustrations, eight four-color illustrations, 269 charts, five pages of bibliography with 72 listings, and a 54 page index that covers both books. Some listings contain as many as 10 references to other medical/dental literature.

Book II contains: 471 pages, including 209 illustrations, six four-color illustrations, and two pages of bibliography.

Dr. Price was a man devoted to the various sciences involved with the subject of health. His extensive studies of his patients' own medical histories, as well as that of three generations of their families, demonstrates his understanding of the genetic factors involved in the immune system and in health. It is only in the last 10 years or so that the real importance of our genetic disposition has become well recognized, but Price demonstrated concern for the issue long ago.

His degrees, honors and affiliations testify further to the versatility of his efforts and the phenomenal range of his thought processes:

WESTON ANDREW VALLEAU PRICE

Doctor of Dental Surgery, University of Michigan
Master of Science Degree, University of Michigan
Certificate of Honor, American Medical Association
Recognition Tribute from the Cleveland Dental Society signed by 28 of its past presidents
Fellow, American College of Dentists
Past President of the Cleveland Dental Society, Northern Ohio State Dental Association and the Ohio State Dental Association
President and Managing Director of the American Dental Association Research Institute for 14 years
Honorary Member, American Academy of Applied Nutrition

Honorary Member, Eugene Field Society
Honorary Member, International College of Dentists
Honorary Member, Mark Twain Society

and a member of the:
American Dental Association
American Association of Applied Science
American Association of Physical Anthropologists
Biological Society of Great Britain
International Association of Dental Research

ABOUT THE USE of ANIMALS in THIS RESEARCH

Some people will criticize the use of animals in this research. It must be remembered that at the time these studies were made such criticism was practically unheard of. However, Price was very conscious of the animals' contribution to society. This is what he had to say:

> *"These researches have required the use of approximately five hundred rabbits a year, for several years; and, for those who would criticize their use, I wish to state that many of these rabbits have in my judgment made a far greater individual contribution and service to the welfare of humanity than hosts of human beings.*
>
> *Rabbits that run wild and are chased by their enemies have not been as well fed and as happily housed, or been privileged to die under chloroform. I have had many patients express their gratitude and confidence by offering themselves for any experiments that I would care to try upon them, if, by so doing, they too could help humanity.*
>
> ***The greatest tragedy that I see in the whole development of this subject in the past has been that humans alone have been used as the experimental material and the experiments have not been properly checked;** for it has been considered that comfort and serviceability were a sure proof of the success of the experiment, entirely misapprehending that a lack of reaction about the tooth, and the consequent comfort, only meant that the quarantine was not in operation and the toxin and bacterial invasion were passing to other parts of the body, there to break down tissue and shorten life."*

TO DO or NOT TO DO ROOT CANAL THERAPY

From all that has been presented in this book, I imagine most readers will conclude that Price was in favor of extracting all root canal filled teeth and would never consider treating one.

You will be pleased to know that is not what he recommended. In spite of Price's 1,174 pages of data that demonstrate the existence of so many documented serious side effects to root canal therapy and the significant role root canal filled teeth play in the creation of degenerative diseases, he stated: *"Don't jump to the conclusion that all root filled teeth should be extracted."* Then he added...

> *"I am not ready to draw the line so rigidly as to state that all root filled teeth should be extracted for every patient or for all patients in any given time, though I do believe there is a limit of safety for all such teeth for each and every patient."*

Time and again he states that the governing factor that must dominate the decision for a dentist or patient as to whether a root canal treatment should be undertaken, or whether a tooth that has a root canal restoration should or should not be retained, depends on that person's defense system and any family genetic problems they may have inherited.

If the individual's immune system is battling one or more degenerative illnesses, or if the patient's parents and grandparents had histories of chronic diseases indicating increased susceptibility, then Price favored avoiding treatment of infected teeth and recommended the removal of any that had received endodontic treatment.

On the other hand, if the patient was in good health and his or her family members were also relatively healthy, this was regarded as an indication that the patient's immune system would apt to be capable of controlling the bacteria involved in root filled teeth.

In fact, Price found that 25 percent of patients with family histories free of degenerative diseases who had excellent immune systems could expect to have and retain root canal fillings and to live without complications arising therefrom through old age. This seems to indicate that these patients' polymorphonuclear white blood cells are standing guard and doing their work of engulfing and destroying invading bacteria.

We now know that the immune system also has T helper and T suppressor cells and that when the system is functioning adequately these cells have a normal ratio between them. Any infection depletes this ratio. Cancer patients have a depletion of the immune system helper cells and have low ratios of 0.6 to 0.8, while those with AIDS can be worse: 0.4 to 0.1.

It should be obvious that keeping root filled teeth, or infection from any source, in someone whose immune system is already compromised by other diseases or injuries is unwise; therefore, it would seem appropriate for such people not to have root canal therapy or retain root filled teeth.

Let me quote another passage from Price's volumes as, by his words, you can sense the depth and extent of his studies and the open-minded clearheadedness with which he viewed the discoveries he had made. He states:

> *"If my interpretation of the preceding researches are correct, there is need for a recasting of the fundamentals for diagnosis, prognosis, and treatment; and I am not unmindful of the tremendous responsibility that I am assuming in suggesting a new alignment of these fundamental principles.*
>
> *It has been because of a recognition of this tremendous responsibility that I have refrained from publishing these data until after I have had a chance to test them out on not a few hundred but on many hundreds of cases, and my presumption and my final willingness to do so are based entirely upon my personal confidence that they are correct.*
>
> *I do not assume that my interpretations are correct in every detail as later information will indicate, but in the light of present knowledge, they seem to me to be the most logical, and I feel it my duty to give them to humanity and the professions in order that others may assist me in correcting and enlarging them as further facts may indicate.*
>
> *I hope to have an opportunity to strengthen or reinterpret with the addition of new data which I am rapidly accumulating. I have no interest or desire that these suggestions shall prevail, except as they may be found to be based upon truth, and he will be my most kind friend who will furnish data to establish their incorrectness."*

Though double blind studies had not yet been established in his time, Price's awareness of inherent problems of misinterpretation caused him to repeat experiments a vast number of times and by different means, using many animals as subjects.

For example, in investigating sterilizing medicaments, Price tested over 100 and did so using a variety of procedures. He stated on a number of occasions that he believed firmly in the accuracy of his deductions but that he welcomed any new developments that would show error or would offer improvement over what he had extrapolated.

In the area of medicaments, some new developments have taken place. Drs. A. Bystrom, R. Claesson, and G. Sundquist, members of the Department of Endodontics and Microbiology at the School of Dentistry, Umei, Sweden, reported in 1985 on the ability of camphorated paramonochlorophenol, camphorated phenol, and calcium hydroxide to kill the bacteria that infect root canals. This information is being presented as none of these three medicaments were mentioned by Price in the over 100 he studied, and they may be an improvement in treatment procedure.

When root canals were treated with camphorated phenol or camphorated paramonochlorophenol, bacteria were found to still be present in 10 of 30 root canals (33 percent). However, with most strains of bacteria, calcium hydroxide was found to kill them in one minute. In samples taken two to four days after the dressings had been removed, bacteria were found in only one of 35 root canals — none when dressings were left for one month.

Here again, it is interesting that Dr. Bystrom and his co-worker researchers found the most resistant (hardest to kill) bacteria were the streptococcus fecalis strain, the very same bacteria species Price found to be the most prevalent — the strain that caused 65 percent of focal infection involvement of glands and tissues of the cases he studied. In general, the streptococcus fecalis species are found in human feces, in the intestines of warm-blooded animals, in urinary infections, in blood and heart lesions of subacute endocarditis cases, and in mild outbreaks of food poisoning.

Price repeatedly stated that he hoped future investigators would find new medicaments or methods to adequately sterilize teeth. The results obtained in the Swedish study were made from culturing the inside of the root canal. In view of the efficiency of calcium hydroxide, it now behooves these investigators or others to take teeth treated in this manner and implant them under the skin of rabbits to determine whether or not the bacteria contained in the dentin tubules are killed by their medications. Such treated teeth could also be sectioned or powdered and cultures attempted in order to investigate the species of bacteria present.

Another new method of sterilizing root canals that should be adequately tested has been reported by Drs. L. Tronstad, Z.P. Yang, M. Trope, F. Barnett and B.F. Hammond, researchers at the University of Pennsylvania School of Dentistry, Department of Endodontics and Microbiology. They developed "controlled release of medicaments in endodontic therapy." The controlled release delivery system comprises a solid inner core matrix that contains the medicament, surrounded by an outer polymeric membrane that is insoluble in body fluids.

The medicaments tested were formocresol, cresatin, parachlor phenol, and quaternary ammonium compound. Young mongrel dogs were used to place root canal treatments and test this new method.

Fresh medicaments on cotton pellets were placed in the pulp chambers of well-prepared and cleansed root canals; others were placed using the controlled release preparation. The formocresol and cresatin in the controlled release trial had no bacteriocidal effect, nor did any of the medicaments on the cotton pellets. Only the quaternary ammonium compound had an effect on bacterial growth after one day in the root canal. This ability to control bacteria continued through the third, seventh and 45th days of the study.

The researchers reported that quaternary ammonium compounds were found to be bacteriocidal for a wide range of organisms including gram positive and negative species, candida albicans, and anaerobic bacteria. They found the test organism streptococcus fecalis, though difficult to kill, was especially promising for research purposes. However, this medicament proved ineffective against mycobacterium tuberculosis, pseudomonas aeriginoza, spores, and most viruses.

It appears that this time release idea of delivering medicaments can open the door to ways that root canals can be adequately sterilized. Fortunately, Dr. Price has provided us with animal study methods to ascertain that ability. Proof of the value and ability of time released medicaments to kill the bacteria that reside in dentin tubules must be determined. To depend on data based on the root canal alone is inadequate.

As mentioned earlier, one other new method of sterilizing root canals is being investigated — that is, the use of lasers. To date, the information from users is enthusiastic but far too little serious research has been completed as of this moment.

Because new methods can possibly solve prevalent root canal treatment problems is no reason for complacency and a do-nothing attitude. In view of the current side effect problems and the role of streptococcus and other oral bacteria in the cause of heart disease; and the fact that the number of deaths from heart disease has increased since Price's time from 10 percent to more than half of all deaths at the current time; and inasmuch as deaths from dental treatment have been considered very rare, the discovery of heart disease transmission from dentin tubules calls upon the dental profession to reassess its role in the appalling number of deaths resulting from this disorder.

It is even more discouraging to realize that one-third of all disease in this country can be either directly or indirectly traced to dental infections. Not only must my profession reappraise its responsibilities, but we have to seriously consider Price's charge that one-third of all of these degenerative diseases can be banished by:

1) Proper nutrition and mastication
2) Proper prophylaxis
3) Proper dental operating procedures

Just when and how these changes are going to take place is a good question. There are two significant pressures that have been known to bring about rapid changes in the thinking of dentists and physicians. The most important one is an enlightened public. Today, with the help of radio and television, public awareness is making for unusually prompt turnarounds in thinking about medical problems.

The other way a change in thinking occurs rapidly is when the individual dentist or physician, or a family member, needs a root canal filling, or already has one, and recovery from a degenerative health problem is not being achieved. At such a time, reassessment of the possibility of the presence of a focal infection assumes urgent importance.

But what if the person ill with a degenerative disease does not recover, or does so only partially after elimination of the focal infection source? We must remember that nutritional deficiencies and excesses can also play a leading role in these illnesses. If both problems have been eliminated and the person remains ill, other sources of infection — bacterial, viral, fungal and parasitic — must be considered. Restoring an ill person to health demands careful consideration of any and every possible contingency.

People do not have to become sick or die from focal infections. However, to stop or prevent their occurrence, the bacteria and their toxins that arise from the dentin tubules or other sources must be eliminated.

It is natural to look upon all of this information negatively. Certainly it is tragic such important discoveries were squelched in the 1920s and 1930s, as by now dentists might have resolved many of the problems that seriously confront us today.

A statement made long ago by the German philosopher, Arthur Schopenhauer, is very appropriate to the root canal side effect issue.

> *"All truth passes through three phases: first it is ridiculed; next it is violently opposed; and finally it is accepted as self-evident."*

Millions of Americans can be spared unspeakable suffering and our country can save billions of dollars when the necessity for the sterilization of root canals and their dentin tubules becomes a reality.

Seeking the new in the old makes good sense when considering the contributions of Weston A. Price, who was certainly an extraordinary dental research specialist — the world's foremost; a true genius who worked relentlessly to alleviate illness and unnecessary death; a man whose every project was based on prevention; and one whose easy and kindly manner made him a true friend and benefactor to mankind.

EPILOGUE

After completing the main chapters of this book about Dr. Price's discoveries of the serious side effects of root canal therapy, galley proofs were sent to several friends and acquaintances for review and comment.

Everyone was shocked to learn of the side effects that can arise from root canals. Many were impressed with the amount of data presented, but some expressed concern that the technical terms would be intimidating to some readers.

The surprise was that non-professional men and women found the book easy to read and comprehend despite the technical names that need to be used for identification purposes. All demonstrated an excellent grasp of what the book is all about.

One person was distressed that dentists don't inform patients that there are alternatives to root canal therapy.

Saving teeth has become such a motivating force that perhaps some dentists do not offer patients a choice. However, I doubt this is a common occurrence. Such an approach never occurred to me in my practice. I always informed patients of the advantages of saving the tooth and, at the same time, the fact that treatment isn't always successful. In other words, they were informed that their options were to extract the tooth or to try and save it.

No longer can doctors insist they know what is best for people and their word is law. People have become very sophisticated about health matters and many realize that they must make the final decision as to what is done to their body and its chemistry. Prevention of illness and disease is largely in the hands of the individual not that of doctors.

One good friend and honest critic, a woman who understands patient responsibility, was disappointed that I hadn't written about the nutritional factors involved in preventing the need of root canal therapy.

In several places throughout the book, I do mention the importance of nutrition but I did not elaborate upon the subject. That was a mistake that I will rectify now in this epilogue.

If the need for root canal treatment is to be prevented, several important factors need to be understood.

The first concerns the fact that almost everyone looks upon tooth decay as a trivial matter. Consequently there is not much concern over whether a tooth has a tiny cavity or a deep one. However, deep cavities lead to the necessity for root canal treatment — which is a very serious matter, certainly not a trifling one.

Though almost everyone is aware that sugar is a factor in tooth decay, very little limiting of sweets in the diet is taking place. In spite of all the other sweeteners now on the market, and there are questions about these as well, the average consumption of sugar is listed as 120 pounds per person per year. That translates into 13 teaspoonsful per person per day.

None of you will admit to using that amount, but a glazed donut has 6 teaspoonsful of sugar, a piece of cake 5, a fig newton 5 (who stops at one), a macaroon 6, a piece of apple pie 12, and à la mode 18. It isn't so much a question of what diet to follow or what foods to eat, but what foods and beverages *not* to consume.

These have been given the commonly used term of "junk foods." It is not only sugar that is a foodless food, but also white flour, refined, highly processed cereals, grain foods vegetable oils; a whole gamut of beverages such as soft drinks, coffee, tea, cocoa, alcoholic drinks, milk (yes, milk), fruit juices (we were meant to chew our food); and the deep fat fried foods and table snacks like fritos, corn and potato chips. Food items fabricated by industrial food manufacturers have become our primary diet problem.

After looking at this list, most people say, "What is there left to eat?" If you are such a person, your diet is most likely highly compromised. What is left of course are all those fresh, natural, nutritious foods that are now available to us year-round in markets all over the country — but were not available 50 years ago.

It is dangerous wishful thinking to rely on toothbrushes, fluorine toothpastes and fluoridated water, and ignore diet.

Dr. Ralph Steinman's research (see Chapter 3) demonstrated how junk foods produce not only a local destructive action on teeth but general body system degradation action as well. Dentists restore diseased teeth quite efficiently but treatment of degenerated body tissues is notably very poor.

Chapter 11 covers the importance of the body's calcium balance, what happens to calcium because of tooth infections, and the crucial relationship of calcium to phosphorus.

Dr. Weston Price, after completing his root canal research, spent nine years traveling the globe investigating the primitive cultural habits of 14 races of people. All primitives he examined had practically no tooth decay, crookedness of teeth, or impacted teeth. They were free of these problems and the degenerative diseases common to us until they were introduced to civilized man's white flour and sugar. In one generation consuming such foods caused them to develop many of the same diseases we experience.

The interesting fact is that although these many diverse tribes of 14 races lived on widely different diets, they universally maintained excellent health until they were introduced to our foods.

So the good news is that you are not locked into any one specific diet as long as man-made items are eliminated. For additional information on prevention, I suggest you refer to the addendum and learn how to obtain Price's book, *Nutrition and Physical Degeneration* — and also see the last pages of this book for information on how to obtain my other book, *"NEW"trition – How to Achieve Optimum Health.*

If you have any root filled teeth in your mouth, you no doubt are disturbed to learn of their side effects. However, I trust that because of this information you will find the long-term effects will prove of great benefit to your health.

Attempt the end and never stand to doubt;
Nothing's so hard, but search will find it out.

– Herrick
Seeke and Finde

ADDENDUM

The Price Pottenger Nutrition Foundation

Those of you who have read the preceding pages of this book will appreciate why Dr. Weston Price was called "The World's Greatest Dentist." No doubt you will also agree that he was a genius.

In view of his wide accomplishments, it is easy to see why he was the most popular speaker of his time at dental, medical and lay group meetings.

Though he became famous for his classic nine year nutritional study of people all over the globe and his highly acclaimed book, *Nutrition and Physical Degeneration*, he is virtually unknown for his root canal research. Now I predict that his fame will be revived and expanded as this previously undisclosed information about his root canal studies reaches the public.

Sometime after Dr. Price's death in 1947, the Price Pottenger Nutrition Foundation was established (P.P.N.F.). The Foundation has two primary functions. The first is to make his book, *Nutrition and Physical Degeneration*, available to anyone interested in the diets of native, primitive and traditional cultures and why what they learned and practiced is so important to our knowledge of nutrition and health. Secondly, P.P.N.F. is the custodian of all the Price research data and memorabilia, which includes over 18,000 photographs of the numerous primitives and animals involved in his root canal research.

Upon the death of Francis M. Pottenger, Jr., M.D., the Foundation also became the custodian of Pottenger's huge research collection. The majority of this data involves Pottenger's 10 year study of cats. Like Price's work, Pottenger's research reveals numerous very basic truths about body chemistry and its relationship to the foods we eat.

This remarkable investigation discloses what happens to cats when they follow a raw rather than cooked meat diet — or raw milk versus pasteurized, evaporated, or sweetened condensed milk.

The startling differences in the animals' health, longevity, and genetic disposition due to the loss of enzymes, vitamins and minerals opens our eyes to some basic causes of degenerative breakdown. Anyone pursuing the quest for optimum nutrition must obtain *Pottenger's Cats — A Study in Nutrition*, as well as Price's book, *Nutrition and Physical Degeneration*, from P.P.N.F.

Over the years, the Foundation has flourished due to the interest of nutrition minded professionals and the public in the contributions these two greats have made in the health field. Under its Executive Director, Pat Connolly, the Foundation has taken on many new responsibilities. One of the most popular is the maintenance of a list of physicians, dentists and other health professionals who are acquainted with nutrition research and apply it in their practices. A call to the Foundation office will secure the name of someone in your area.

Of interest along these lines is a report in the *New England Journal of Medicine* from the Eisenberg Group on the subject of alternative medicine. This survey indicated that one third of the people in the United States use alternative medicine. 14.7 billion dollars was expended in 1990 and only 10 percent tell their doctors they are using any of these "unconventional" techniques.

All professionals who become P.P.N.F. members are asked to submit background information about their practice and interests in order for their names to be included on the referral list. Dentists who have a nutritional background are in demand. The Foundation is also seeking the names of dental members who are practicing amalgam free dentistry, and those who understand the side effect dangers of root canal therapy and follow the extraction protocol.

If you are impressed with what Dr. Weston Price and Dr. Francis Pottenger have done for humanity and are interested in learning more, call P.P.N.F. at 1-800-FOODS 4 U (1-800-366-3748) and arrange for membership in this vital organization which welcomes both the lay person and the professional.

The benefits of membership are impressive: twenty-first century nutrition information, a quarterly journal, an extensive library of nutritional books, and numbers of additional publications are available for sale. When you call, request the book list catalogue. Members receive a 10 percent discount on books published by the Foundation and, from time to time, meetings and seminars are conducted by leading health practitioners.

You often hear the remark, "It is more beneficial to give than to receive." This is one of those instances when the benefits one receives far exceeds what is given.

Regarding the Bibliography of the Two Weston Price Volumes

A large number of the Dr. Weston Price research discoveries were from original work that he created and developed. However, a fair amount of it was also stimulated by the work of the 60 members who were the key professionals involved in the management of the Research Institute of the American Dental Association (A.D.A.) that Price directed. This research division of the A.D.A. had the best research workers, the finest equipment, and the most complete dental library in the world.

In the view of the prevalence of tooth decay and gum diseases in the world and their relationship to the cause of numerous other serious body ailments the purpose of the Research Institute was to investigate the reasons for the occurrences of these diseases and their prevention.

The 60 Research Institute scientists contributed much to the basic background involved in the Dr. Price investigations.

In addition, Dr. Price was an avid follower of the scientific literature. His two books about root canal therapy contained a bibliography listing of 86 references. Rather than list all of the 86 but to give you an appreciation of the scope of their coverage, listed below are 20 of his references,

In my own efforts to obtain information that substantiated or disproved the Dr. Price studies a considerable amount of data was reviewed. The associated research endeavors mentioned in this book are contained in my bibliography.

Partial Bibliography of Dr. Weston Price

Mayo, Charles H.: Mouth infection as a source of systemic disease. A.M.A. Jnl., LXIII, 1914, 2025-2026. Disc. 2029-2032. Amer. D. Jnl., XII, 1914-15, 407-412, 2 illus. Brit. D. Jnl., XXXVI, 1915, 1-4.

The relation of mouth conditions to general health (re care of school children). N.D.A. Jnl., VI, 1919, 505-512.

Hunter, W.: Coming of age of oral sepsis. Brit. M.J. 1:859, June 11, '21.

Oral sepsis as a cause of disease. London, Paris, N.Y. and Melbourne: Cassel & Co., Ltd. 1911.

The role of sepsis and antisepsis in medicine and the importance of oral sepsis as its chief cause. Register, LXV, 1911, 579-596. Abstract.

Oral sepsis in relationship to "Septic Anemia." Brit. D. Jnl., XXXV, 1914, 161. Disc. 161-163. Record, XXXIV, 1914, 144. Disc. 144-146. Selected.

Billings, Frank: Focal Infection. New York: D. Appleton & Co., 1917, 1918.

Mouth infection as a source of systemic disease. Pacific D. Gaz., XXV, 1917, 261-262. Selected

Dublin, Louis I.: Incidence of heart disease in community. Nation's Health 4:453-456, Aug. '22.

Rosenau, E.C.: Mouth infection as a source of systemic disease. A.M.A. Jnl., LXIII, 1914, 2027. Disc. 2029-2032. Summary, XXXV, 1915, 4-6.
Elective localization of the streptococcus from a case of pulpitis, dental neuritis and myositis. Ortho. Int. Jnl. II, 1916, 713-725, 16 illus., 1 table. Cosmos, LIX, 1917, 561-562. Abstract
The relation of dental infection to systemic disease. Allied XII, 1917, 400. Abstract. Cosmos, LIX, 1917; 485-491, 2 tables. Pacific D. Gaz., XXV, 1917, 612-620, 2 tables. Selected. Register, LXXI, 1917, 286-289. Abstract.
The pathogenesis of focal infection. Cosmos, LX, 1918, 303. Abstract, N.D.S. Jnl., V, 1918, 113-124, 6 illus.
Focal infection with special reference to oral sepsis. Minneapolis Dist. D. Jnl., II, Dec., 1919-20, 3-5.
Studies on elective localization: Focal infection with special reference to oral sepsis. N.D.A. Jnl., VI, 1919, 983-1023, 46 illus. Disc. 1024-1029. Portrait, 982. Research Jnl., I, 1919, 205-267, 1 illus., 2 tables, 9 plates. Disc. pp. lxxii-lxxxi, 6 illus. Comment, 519-522
Elective localation and focal infection from oral sepsis. Register, LXXIII, 1919, 557-567. Abstracts. Brit. D. Jnl., XLI, 1920, 223-224. Abstract.
Elective localization of bacteria following various methods of inoculation, and production of nephritis by devitalization and infection of teeth in dogs. J. Lab. & Clin. Med. 7:707-722, Sept. '22.
and Meisser, J.G.: Nephritis and urinary calculi after production of chronic foci of infection, preliminary report. J.A.M.A. 78:266-267, Jan. 28, '22.

Olitsky, P.K., and Gates, F.L.: Methods for isolation of filter-passing anaerobic organisms from human nasopharyngeal secretions. J.A.M.A. 78-1020-1022, April 8, '22.

Libman, E.: Characterization of various forms of endocarditis. J.A.M.A., Vol. 80,No. 12.

Goadby, K.W.: Diagnosis of latent infection about the jaws. J.A.D.A. Part I, May, 1922, p. 371; Part II, June 1922, p. 504.
Streptococcal infections arising from mouth. J. State Med. 30:415-423, Oct. '22.

George E. Meinig, D.D.S. Bibliography

The following articles published since Dr. Price's time contain information that relates in some way to his research. Many were sighted during the presentation of the text material.

McKay, G.S.: The pattern of bacterial invasion of carious dentin. Jr. Dent. Research. No. 6, Vol. 48, 1969.

Fabricius, Lars; Dahleu, Gunnar; Öhman, Alf E; Moller, Ake J.R.: Predominant indigenous oral bacteria isolated from infected root canals after varied times of closure. Dept. Oral Microbiology and Oral Diagnosis. Union of Gothenbury, Sweden.

Torabinejad, M; Kahn, Henry; Boukes, Donna: Isopropyl cyanoacrylate as a root canal sealer. Jr. of Endodontics.

Barnett, F.; Trope, M.; Krestool, D.; Tronstad, L.: Suitability of controlled release delivery system for root canal disinfection.

Cheraskin, E.; Ringsdorf, Jr.: 1. Two-hour post prandial blood glucose frequency distribution. Jnl. Oral Med., Jan. 1968, Vol. 23.

Cheraskin, E.; Ringsdorf. Jr.: II. Causes of periopical pathosis and two-hour post prandial blood glucose. Jnl. Oral Med., April 1968, Vol. 23.

Cheraskin, E.; Ringsdorf, Jr.: The biology of the endodontic patient: III.Variability in periapical healing and blood glucose. Jnl. of Oral Medicine, Jan. 1986, Vol. 23.

Kahn, Henry: Making endodontics a little easier. Dental Clinics of North America, Oct. 1984, Vol. 28.

Segall, R.O.; del Rio, Carlos E.: Cavitational bone defect: A diagnostic challenge. Jnl. of Endodontics, Aug. 1991.

Rotner, E.J.; Langer, B.; Evins, M.L.: Alveolar cavitational osteopathosis manifestations of an infectious process and its implication in the causation of chronic pain. Jnl. of Periodontology, Oct. 1986.

Bouquot, J.E.; Roberts, A.M.; Person, P.; Christian, J.: Neuralgia-inducing cavitational osteonecrosis (NICO) oral surgery. Oral Med., Oral Path, 1992;73

Bouquot, J.E.: More about neuralgia-inducing cavitational osteonecrosis (NICO) oral surg. Oral Med., Oral Path., Sept. 1992.

Fischer, M.H., Professor Physiology: Book — Death and dentistry. Charles C. Thomas Pub., Springfield, IL 1940.

Sundqvist G.: Bacteriological studies of necrotic dental pulps. Umea University Odontological Dissertation no. 7. Univ. of Umea, Sweden, 1976.

Möller, AJR; Fabricius, L.; Dahlen, G.; Öhman, E.E.; Hevoen, G.: Influence on periapical tissues of indigenous oral bacteria and necrotic pulp tissue. An experimental study in monkeys. Scand. J. Dent. Res. 1981, 89:475-84.

Uchin, R.A.; Parris, L.: Antibacterial activity of endodontic medications after varying time intervals within the root canal. Oral Surg. 1963, 16:608-12.

Treanor, H.T.: Bactericidal efficiency of intracanal medications. Oral Surg. 1972. 33:791-6.

Tronstad L.; Yang, A.P.; Trope, M.; Barnett, F.; Hammond, B.: Controlled release of medicaments in endodontic therapy. Endod Dent Traumatol, 1985. 1:130-4.

Engström, B.; Spangbert, L.: Studies on root canal medicaments. 1. Cytoloxic effect of root canal antiseptics. Acid Odontol Scand. 1967, 25:77-84.

Spangbert, L.; Engström, B.: Studies on root canal medicaments. 11. Antimicrobal effect of root canal medicaments. Odontol Revy 1968, 2:187-95.

Möller, AJR: Microbiological examination of root canals and peripical tissues of human teeth. Thesis. Odontol Tidskr (Special Issue) 1966, 74:1-380.

Cvek, M.: Treatment of nonvital permanent incisors with calcium hydroxide. 1. Follow-up periapical repair and apical closure of immature roots. Ondont Revy 1972, 23:27-44.

Bystrom, A.; Claesson, R.; Sundqvist, G.: The antibacterial effect of camphorated paramonochlorphenol, camphorated phenol and calcium hydroxide in the treatment of infected root canals. Endod Dent Traumatol 1985, 1:170

Tronstad, L.; Andreasen, JO; Hasselgren, G.; Kristerson, L; Riis 1. pH changes in dental tissues following root canal filing with calcium hydroxide. An experimental study in monkeys. J Endod 1981, 7:17-21.

Gordon, W.; Barnett, F.; Trope, M.; Tronstad, L.: Tissue response to a quaternary ammonium compound in a controlled release vehicle. Abstract no. 559. IADR 1986.

Baumgartner, JC; Heggers, JP; Harrison, JW: The incidence of bacteremias related to endodontic procedures. 1. Non surgical endodontics. J. Endodon 1976, 2:135-40.

Beechen, II; Laston, OJ; Barbarino, VE: Transitory bacteremia as related to the operation of vital pulpotomy. Oral Surg 1956, 9:902-5.

Klotz, MD; Gerstein, JH; Bahn, AN: Bacteremia after topical use of prednisone in infected pulps. J Am Dent Assoc 1965, 71:871-5.

Bhaskar, SN: Periapical lesion-types., incidence and clinical features. Oral Surg 1966, 21:659.

Stern, MH: Cell-mediated immune response in human apical granulomas. (Abstract). J Dent Res 1979, 50:130.

Winslow, MB; Millstone, SH: Bacteremia after prophylaxis. J Periodontal 1965, 36:371-4.

Scopp, IW; Orvietto, LD: Gingival degerming by povidone-iodine irrigation: bacteremia reduction in extraction procedures. J Am Dent Assoc 1971, 83:1294-6.

McGowan, DA; Hardie JM: Production of bacterial endocarditis in prepared rabbits by oral manipulation. Br Dent J 1974, 137:129-91.

Bahn, S:; Ross, D; Biencevenga, G; Bahn, AN: Experimental endocarditis induced by oral streptococci. J Dent Res IADR Abstract 1974, #69.

Afterward

I hope exposé information about the long lost and buried Dr. Price research disclosures has proved helpful to you and your family. ***Should you have had an experience with root canals that you feel will be of importance for others to learn about, please drop me a line concerning the occurrence.***

Dr. George
In care of — BION PUBLISHING
323 East Matilija Street, 110-151A
Ojai, California 93023

ABOUT THAT OTHER BOOK OF MINE.. "NEW"TRITION — How to Achieve Optimum Health

It received the Benjamin Franklin Finalist Award for Achievement in the Health Field.

• *"What makes this book so interesting for the average reader is that these are not dry, lengthy chapters on the science of nutrition. These are direct answers to questions readers ask about health and related problems. For years, Dr. Meinig's writing has been ahead of his peers."* Fred Volz, Editor & Publisher

• *"He brings nutrition up to date showing the importance of minerals is equal to that of vitamins, and emphasizes how crucial the balance of minerals is to human health. "* Mary Jane Hungerford, Ph.D.

• *"The excellent basic coverage of a wide range of subjects shows Dr. Meinig's extensive background and experience to be the reason his words so well clarify the confusion of data being presented."...* Bob McEntee, Scientist

Please see the back of this page for order information and a special discount offer.

Index

D

E

F

R

S

T

U

V

W

X